NEURO-MUSCULOSKELETAL CLINICAL TESTS
A Clinician's Guide

Richard Day BSc(Hons) MCSP
*Lecturer, School of Healthcare Studies,
Cardiff University, Cardiff, UK*

John Fox MSc MCSP
*Lecturer, School of Healthcare Studies,
Cardiff University, Cardiff, UK*

Graeme Paul-Taylor BSc(Hons) MCSP MACP
*Physiotherapy Practitioner, Cwm Taf NHS Trust, Prince
Charles Hospital, Merthyr Tydfil, UK*

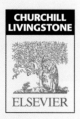

CHURCHILL
LIVINGSTONE

ELSEVIER

Edinburgh   London   New York   Oxford   Philadelphia
St Louis   Sydney   Toronto   2009

CHURCHILL
LIVINGSTONE
ELSEVIER

First published 2009

ISBN 978-0-443-06945-1

British Library Cataloguing in Publication Data
A catalogue record for this book is available from the British Library

Library of Congress Cataloging in Publication Data
A catalog record for this book is available from the Library of Congress

Notice
Neither the Publisher nor the Authors assume any responsibility for any loss or injury and/or damage to persons or property arising out of or related to any use of the material contained in this book. It is the responsibility of the treating practitioner, relying on independent expertise and knowledge of the patient, to determine the best treatment and method of application for the patient.

The Publisher

1005 68 70 4 2

The publisher's policy is to use paper manufactured from sustainable forests

Printed in China

NEUROMUSCULOSKELETAL CLINICAL TESTS

09

For Elsevier:

Commissioning Editor: Rita Demetriou-Swanwick
Development Editor: Veronika Watkins
Project Manager: Gail Wright
Design Direction: Erik Bigland
Illustration Manager: Bruce Hogarth

Contents

Preface

Clinical tests are designed to identify potential neuromusculoskeletal problems or pathologies. One issue that arises during the education of healthcare professionals at an undergraduate and a postgraduate level is that students have difficulty in applying the theory of a clinical test to the practical application and interpretation of the test. The concept of this publication is to provide developing clinicians with the necessary theoretical and practical information for a clinical test in a clear and standardized format that enables the clinician to identify which part of the information about a clinical test they require. There are three distinct sections to each test. First, each test has an introduction, explaining what the test is designed to test and its potential mechanism. Second, each test has a clearly laid out procedure divided into the patient's and the clinician's role during the test. These are supported by figures illustrating a specific aspect of the test. Third, each test has a findings section that states the positive and negative findings of each test. In addition to these three sections, some clinical tests have a table listing the sensitivity and specificity values of the test. Sensitivity and specificity tables were included for clinical tests where literature on the values was identified. The concept of sensitivity and specificity is discussed on page xi.

One considerable challenge in preparing this text was that throughout the literature there is a wide variety of information supplied regarding each clinical test. Some existing texts provide information on the procedure of a clinical test but fail to state clearly the possible findings, while others fail to provide adequate explanation of the procedure of the test. Similarly, there is considerable controversy regarding different procedures and interpretation of tests and occasionally wide variants or refinements of the same test. This mix of evidence provided challenges in the standardization of each test and also the ability to provide evidence-based references for the introduction, procedure and findings.

Each test, therefore, is based on a consensus of identified articles, key texts and clinical experience. It was our decision to format the book in this amalgamation of evidence style rather than disrupt the benefit of the standardization of the text. The literature used can be identified in the bibliography and further reading sections at the end of each chapter. The literature used to formulate the sensitivity and specificity tables is presented in a pure evidence-based format and is referenced accordingly.

Another challenge identified was that trying to locate a test in an index system without knowing the name of the test proved difficult. One benefit of this book is that the index system enables the reader to identify the clinical tests in a number of ways. The clinician may require a full range of tests to assess a particular joint; for example, the knee joint. If requiring ligament integrity tests of the knee specifically, these also can be identified via the index system. If the clinician requires a test for a specific ligament, for example the anterior cruciate ligament of the knee, all clinical tests designed to test this specific ligament are indexed under 'anterior cruciate ligament integrity'. Finally, clinical tests are indexed by their commonly used names. This enables the clinician to access the necessary information within this publication.

The content of this publication provides information that is relevant for both the undergraduate and the experienced clinician. The undergraduate will benefit from the clear layout of each test, the index system and the carefully selected range of tests designed to provide an adequate but not overwhelming selection. The experienced clinician will benefit from the ability to identify variations of clinical tests and the additional sensitivity and specificity values provided for many of the tests, providing evidence-based practice that is easily applied in the clinical environment. Furthermore, the experienced clinician can use the sensitivity and specificity tables to provide useful links to literature which may provide further professional development and perhaps generate ideas for departmental training.

Richard Day
John Fox
Graeme Paul-Taylor

Cardiff 2009

Acknowledgements

We wish to thank our colleagues who have supported us through the writing of this publication and our family and friends who have helped carry us through numerous challenges along the way. We would also like to thank Anita Holmes, Nicholas Howell and Timothy Sharp for their assistance in being willing subjects for the figures. Finally, we wish to thank the staff at Elsevier who have provided endless encouragement and support through the writing process.

Sensitivity and specificity

Clinical tests are used to determine if a patient has a certain disease or a specific pathology. For example, McMurray's test is designed to test the integrity of the menisci within the knee joint. The procedure of the test involves the clinician positioning the knee joint and applying a dynamic compression movement of the tibial and femoral condyles to try to 'catch' a torn piece of cartilage from the meniscus. If a tear of the cartilage is present, you would expect the test to produce an audible 'click' or 'pop', together with reported pain from the patient. In a perfect world this creates a simple choice of results: either the test is negative – i.e., the meniscus is intact – or the test is positive – i.e., the meniscus has been torn. Not all tests are 100% accurate, however: the majority of clinical tests can fail to identify a positive or a negative result. This creates four possible combinations of results for all clinical tests; let's use the McMurray test as an example:

True positive: The patient does have a torn meniscus and the clinical test is a positive result.

False positive: The patient does not have a torn meniscus but the clinical test is a positive result.

True negative: The patient does not have a torn meniscus and the clinical test is a negative result.

False negative: The patient does have a torn meniscus but the clinical test is a negative result.

Let us consider a population of 20 subjects (Fig. 0.1), where 8 of these subjects have a meniscal tear (sad faces) and the remaining 12 subjects do not have a meniscal tear (happy faces).

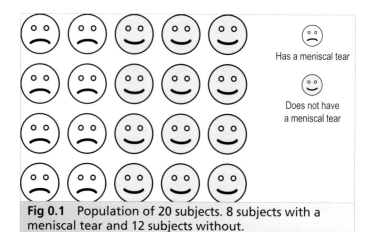

Fig 0.1 Population of 20 subjects. 8 subjects with a meniscal tear and 12 subjects without.

Now, let us imagine the McMurray's test is applied to all 20 subjects and analyse the obtained results (Fig. 0.2).

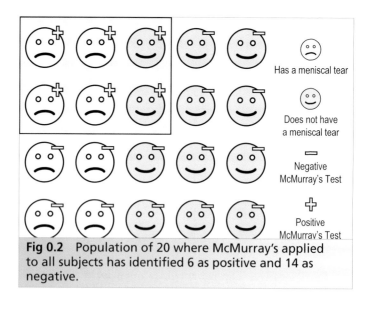

Fig 0.2 Population of 20 where McMurray's applied to all subjects has identified 6 as positive and 14 as negative.

McMurray's test has correctly identified 4 subjects with a torn meniscus (true positives).

McMurray's test has missed 4 subjects with a torn meniscus (false negatives).

McMurray's test has correctly identified 10 subjects do not have a torn meniscus (true negatives).

McMurray's test has incorrectly identified 2 subjects do have a torn meniscus when in fact they do not (false positives).

The true and false positive and true and false negative subjects in our population of 20 enable us to calculate how good the McMurray's test is at correctly identifying that a subject has a torn meniscus; this is known as the *sensitivity* of the test. Also we can calculate how good the McMurray's test is at correctly identifying that a subject does not have a torn meniscus; this is known as the *specificity* of the test. Therefore, the *sensitivity* of a test refers to how good the test is at identifying that pathology is present. This can be expressed as a simple equation:

$$\frac{True\ positives}{(True\ positives\ +\ False\ negatives)}$$

For the McMurray's example, the test has correctly identified 4 out of 8 subjects with a torn meniscus (true positives = 4), and incorrectly identified 4 subjects without a torn meniscus as positive (false positives = 4).

$$\frac{4}{(4\ +\ 4)} = 0.50$$

Expressed as a percentage, in this example, McMurray's test has a *sensitivity* of 50%.

Similarly, the *specificity* of a test refers to how good the test is at identifying that pathology is not present. This can also be expressed as a simple equation:

$$\frac{True\ negative}{(True\ negative\ +\ False\ positive)}$$

For the McMurray's example, the test has correctly identified 10 out of 12 subjects with a torn meniscus (true negatives = 10), and incorrectly identified 2 subjects with a torn meniscus as negative (false positives = 2).

$$\frac{10}{(10\ +\ 2)} = 0.833r$$

Expressed as a percentage, in this example, McMurray's test has a *specificity* of 83%.

Sensitivity and specificity values can assist the clinician in understanding how good the clinical test is at doing what it is supposed to do. A highly sensitive test (e.g., 99%) is very good at identifying that a patient has the pathology, and likewise a highly specific test (e.g., 99%) is very good at identifying that a patient does not have the pathology. Reviewing the above example, it appears that McMurray's test is much better at identifying subjects who do not have a meniscal tear rather than those that do.

A clinician should consider the sensitivity and specificity values of a test when using the test in clinical practice. Taking a test result on face value may lead the clinician to formulate a wrong diagnosis on the basis of a test which may have poor sensitivity or specificity. The clinician should always consider the results of a clinical test against other presenting information from the patient.

Within this publication we have attempted to collate sensitivity and specificity values from a range of literature for the corresponding clinical tests. The literature identified falls into two categories. First, individual studies that have investigated the sensitivity and specificity of a single test or a range of clinical tests, where the authors perform an experimental study, for example, a correlation design study which compares a clinical test against a recognized 'gold standard' such as MRI scan or arthroscopy. Second, systematic reviews or meta-analyses, where the authors perform a search of recognized databases and select individual experimental studies that investigated the sensitivity and specificity of a clinical test. Articles that meet the stated inclusion and exclusion criteria are then analysed for their sensitivity and specificity values. This process of collecting a group of studies improves the overall validity of the findings.

Bibliography and Further Reading

Grove S 2007 Statistics for health care research. Saunders Elsevier, St Louis, MO

Loong T 2003 Understanding sensitivity and specificity with the right side of the brain. British Medical Journal 327(7417): 716–719

The cervical and thoracic spine

SPURLING'S TEST

Spurling's test is designed to test for possible encroachment of a structure into the foraminal canal, and thus possible signs of peripheral nerve entrapment/pathology in the cervical spine. This test is also known as the 'compression test'. The procedure involves asking the patient to side flex their cervical spine, which closes down the size of the intervertebral foramen on that side. The clinician applies a direct gentle pressure to the top of the patient's head, which decreases the intervertebral foramen further. An expected positive response from this test is the reproduction of the patient's symptoms, or production of possible nerve entrapment pathology symptoms such as referral of pain or sensation changes into the corresponding arm.

PROCEDURE
   Patient: The patient is positioned in sitting, with their cervical spine side flexed to the affected side.
   Clinician: The clinician stands behind the patient and applies a gentle downwards pressure to the patient's head (Fig. 1.1). The clinician notes the response from the patient and continues to test the other side.

FINDINGS
   Positive result: A reproduction of the patient's pain/symptoms in the cervical spine and/or corresponding upper limb may suggest potential peripheral nerve entrapment in the cervical spine.

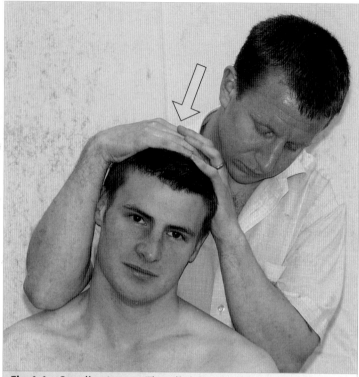

Fig 1.1 Spurling's test. The clinician applies a gentle compressive force to the top of the patient's head while the patient's cervical spine is positioned in side flexion.

Negative result: There will be no reproduction of the patient's symptoms and no referral of symptoms into the patient's corresponding upper limb.

Table 1.1 Sensitivity and specificity values of Spurling's test

Author	Aim of study	Design	Sensitivity	Specificity
Rubinstein et al (2007)	Assessment of the diagnostic accuracy of provocative tests of the neck for diagnosis of cervical radiculopathy	Systematic review of six studies that met selection criteria	Ranged from 50 to 90%	Ranged from 86 to 100%
Tong et al (2002)	To determine the sensitivity and specificity of Spurling's test for cervical radiculopathy	Correlation of 224 subjects' Spurling's test findings with electro diagnosis findings	30%	93%

WRIGHT'S MANOEUVRE

Wright's manoeuvre is designed to test for potential signs of thoracic outlet syndrome. This test is also known as 'Allen's test' or 'Allen's manoeuvre'. The procedure involves positioning the patient's cervical spine and shoulder complex in such a way as to try to occlude nerves and possible blood vessels within the brachial plexus entering the upper limb. Shoulder abduction and lateral rotation may lead to potential compression of the brachial plexus between the anterior aspect of the shoulder joint and surrounding soft tissues. Because of possible vascular occlusion, the radial pulse may be taken both prior to adopting the testing position and during the test. If positive, the radial pulse may feel weaker or absent in the testing position. Asking the patient to breathe in fully may also act to compress tissues further within the costoclavicular region, as full chest expansion decreases the size of the cervicoaxillary canal. An expected positive response from this test may include an absence or weakening of the radial pulse and/or reproduction of the patient's symptoms.

PROCEDURE

Patient: The patient is positioned in sitting, with their cervical spine rotated away from the arm to be tested. The shoulder is positioned in 90° abduction and full lateral rotation; the elbow is positioned in 90° flexion.

Clinician: The clinician is standing behind the patient. The clinician tests the patient's radial pulse prior to the positioning of the upper limb and tests during positioning (Fig. 1.2). The clinician also notes any reproduction of symptoms.

FINDINGS

Positive result: An absence or change in the radial pulse may suggest a degree of compression of the arteries entering the upper limb. Reproduction of the patient's pain or other symptoms, or sensory disturbances, for example, onset of pins and needles or tingling, may suggest compression/stretch of the nervous tissue of the brachial plexus.

Negative result: There will be no change in the radial pulse and no reproduction of the patient's symptoms.

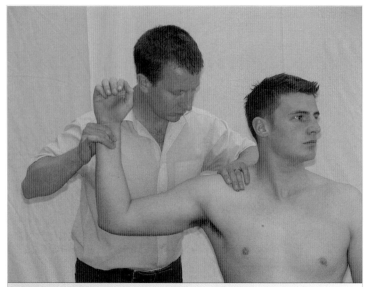

Fig 1.2 Wright's manoeuvre. The clinician takes the patient's pulse while in the test position.

ELEVATED ARM STRESS TEST

The elevated arm stress test (EAST) is designed to test for potential signs of thoracic outlet syndrome. The procedure involves positioning both the patient's shoulders into abduction and full lateral rotation, with the elbows positioned in 90° flexion. The patient opens and closes their hands for 3 minutes. Bilateral shoulder abduction and lateral rotation may lead to potential compression of the brachial plexus between the anterior aspect of the shoulder joint and surrounding soft tissues. Because of possible vascular occlusion, the radial pulse is taken prior to adopting the testing position and during the test. If positive, the radial pulse may feel weaker or absent during the application of the testing position. An expected positive response from this test may include an absence or weakening of the radial pulse and/or reproduction of the patient's symptoms.

PROCEDURE

Patient: The patient is positioned in sitting, with their cervical spine in a neutral position. Both shoulders are positioned in 90° abduction and full lateral rotation; the elbows are positioned into 90° flexion (Fig. 1.3).

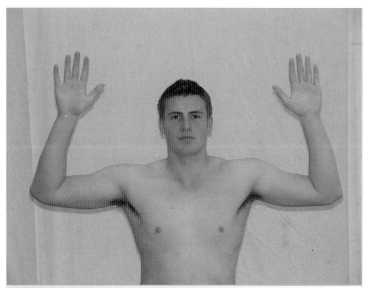

Fig 1.3 Elevated arm stress test. Starting position for the test.

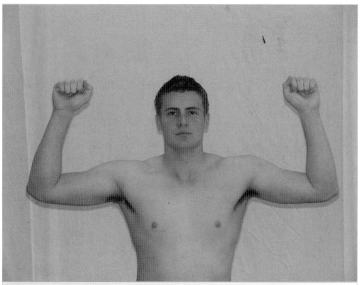

Fig 1.4 Elevated arm stress test. The patient opens and closes their hands for 3 minutes.

Clinician: The clinician is standing in front of the patient and asks the patient to open and close their hands for 3 minutes (Fig. 1.4). The clinician tests the patient's radial pulse prior to the positioning of the upper limb and tests it during/after positioning. The clinician also notes any reproduction of symptoms.

FINDINGS

Positive result: A change in the radial pulse may suggest a degree of compression of the arteries entering the upper limb. Reproduction of the patient's pain or other symptoms or sensory disturbances, for example, onset of pins and needles or tingling, may suggest compression/stretch of the nervous tissue within the brachial plexus.

Negative result: There will be no change in the radial pulse and no reproduction of the patient's symptoms.

REFERENCES

Rubinstein S, Pool J, van Tulder M et al 2007 A systematic review of the diagnostic accuracy of provocative tests of the neck for diagnosing cervical radiculopathy. European Spine Journal 16(3): 307–319

Tong H, Haig A, Yamakawa K 2002 The Spurling test and cervical radiculopathy. Spine 27(2): 156–159

BIBLIOGRAPHY AND FURTHER READING

Magee D 2008 Orthopedic physical assessment, 5th edn. Saunders Elsevier, St Louis, MO

Norris C 2005 Sports injuries diagnosis and management, 3rd edn. Butterworth-Heinemann, Edinburgh

The shoulder

EMPTY CAN TEST

The empty can test is designed to test for impingement and/ or supraspinatus weakness of the shoulder; it may also aid in the identification of other rotator cuff disease/pathology. This test is also known as 'Jobe's position test' and the 'supraspinatus muscle strength test'. The procedure of the test involves placing the shoulder joint into flexion in the scapula plane and medial rotation with the elbow extended, appearing as if emptying a can. The clinician then manually loads the arm. This action is thought to mechanically load the supraspinatus muscle and potentially compress or load the soft tissues within the subacromial space. An expected positive response from this test is to identify muscle weakness and/or reproduce the patient's pain. There is currently an increasing use of the 'full can test'; this is identical in application except that the patient's arm is in full supination.

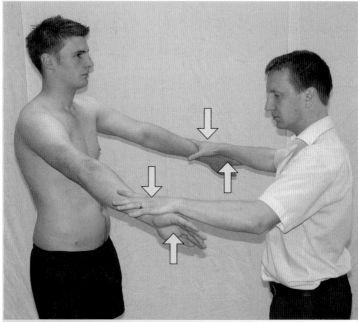

Fig 2.1 Empty can test. The patient attempts to resist the clinician's downwards pressure.

PROCEDURE

Patient: The patient is positioned in standing. The shoulder is flexed in the scapula plane between 40° and 70°, full medial rotation. The elbow is extended and the wrist fully pronated.

Clinician: The clinician is standing in front of the patient, applying a downwards resistance at the patient's elbow or wrist. The clinician may test both shoulders simultaneously to assess for differences (Fig. 2.1).

FINDINGS

Positive result: Pain reported on the anterolateral aspect of the shoulder may suggest impingement. A 'giving way' of the affected limb may suggest either pain inhibition or a full thickness tear in the rotator cuff, predominantly the supraspinatus muscle. A slow lowering of the affected arm on application of the resistance may suggest weakness in the rotator cuff muscles or a partial tear, or demonstrate pain inhibition.

Negative result: There is no reproduction of pain or evidence of muscle weakness.

Table 2.1 Sensitivity and specificity values of the empty can test

Author	Aim of study	Design	Sensitivity	Specificity
Leroux et al (1995)	To determine the diagnostic value of clinical tests for shoulder impingement	Correlation of 55 subjects' preoperative test findings with open surgery and arthroscopy	86%	50%
Park et al (2005)	To determine the diagnostic accuracy of clinical tests for the different degrees of subacromial impingement syndrome	Correlation of 552 subjects' preoperative test findings with arthroscopic findings	44.1%	89.5%

INFRASPINATUS MUSCLE STRENGTH TEST

The infraspinatus muscle strength test is designed to test the integrity of the lateral rotators of the shoulder. The procedure of the test involves applying isometric resistance to the outside of the subject's wrists, against the patient's efforts to laterally rotate. This resistance predominantly loads the infraspinatus muscle; however, other lateral rotators will also contribute to this action. An expected positive response from the test is to demonstrate muscle weakness and/or reproduce the patient's pain.

PROCEDURE
Patient: The patient is positioned in standing. Their shoulder is in slight flexion with the elbow in 90° of flexion and the wrist in the mid position.

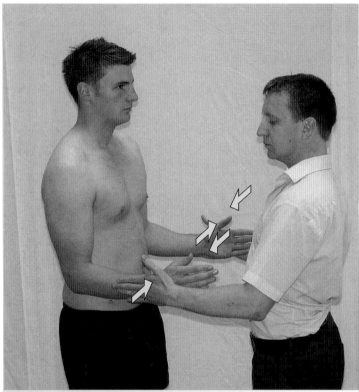

Fig 2.2 Infraspinatus muscle strength test. The patient attempts to resist the clinician's inward pressure.

Clinician: The clinician is standing to the front of the patient, applying an inward resistance to the outside of the patient's wrists. The clinician asks the patient to push outwards, against the applied resistance. The clinician may test both shoulders simultaneously to assess for differences (Fig. 2.2).

FINDINGS

Positive result: An inability of the patient to resist the clinician's applied force may suggest a rupture of the infraspinatus tendon. If considerable pain is present this result may also be due to pain inhibition. If a resistance is present but there is a reduced strength observed this may suggest a partial tear or pain inhibition. Where there is an ability to resist the applied force but the patient complains of pain during the activity this may suggest a tendon- or muscle-based pathology (i.e. tendinopathy).

Negative result: No reproduction of pain or evidence of muscle weakness.

Table 2.2 Sensitivity and specificity values of the infraspinatus muscle strength test

Author	Aim of study	Design	Sensitivity	Specificity
Park et al (2005)	To determine the diagnostic accuracy of clinical tests for the different degrees of subacromial impingement syndrome	Correlation of 552 subjects' preoperative test findings with arthroscopic findings	41.6%	90.1%

EXTERNAL ROTATION LAG SIGN

The external rotation lag sign is designed to test the integrity of the supraspinatus and infraspinatus muscles as part of the rotator cuff. This test is also known as the 'lag sign'. The procedure of the test involves the clinician positioning the patient into full passive lateral rotation of the glenohumeral joint. The clinician instructs the patient to try and hold this position. A rupture or weakness of supraspinatus and/or infraspinatus results in the patient's inability to hold this position; this is demonstrated by a loss of the full laterally rotated position. The degree of drop or loss is known as the lag. An expected positive response from the test is to demonstrate muscle weakness.

PROCEDURE

Patient: The patient is positioned in sitting or standing. The shoulder is positioned into full lateral rotation assisted by the clinician, elbow in 90° flexion.

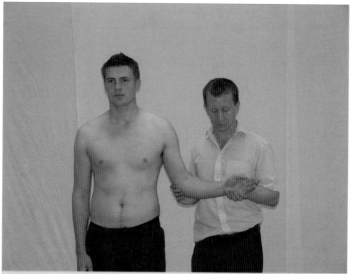

Fig 2.3   External rotation lag sign. The clinician assists the patient into full shoulder external rotation and asks the patient to hold this position.

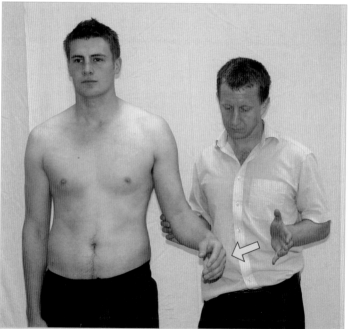

Fig 2.4   External rotation lag sign. A positive lag sign as the arm drops in and forwards.

Clinician: The clinician is standing to the side of the patient. The clinician assists in positioning the patient's shoulder into full lateral rotation (Fig. 2.3), asks the patient to try and hold the position, and releases the arm (Fig. 2.4).

FINDINGS

Positive result: An inability of the patient to hold the required position with a complete lag or dropping of the arm back to a neutral position may suggest a substantial rupture of one or both muscles. A slight lag or loss of position may indicate a partial tear or muscle weakness.

Negative result: No lag present on testing.

LIFT OFF TEST

The lift off test is designed to test the integrity of the subscapularis muscle as part of the rotator cuff. This test is also known as 'Gerber's lift off test'. The procedure of the test involves an isometric hold of the patient's hand away from their back in a position of full medial rotation of the shoulder. This position of maximum medial rotation predominantly loads the subscapularis muscle. An expected positive response is the inability of the patient to maintain this position, suggesting muscle weakness with or without pain.

PROCEDURE

Patient: The patient is positioned in standing. Their affected arm is assisted by the clinician into shoulder extension and maximal shoulder medial rotation so that the patient's hand is adjacent to their lumbar spine.

Clinician: The clinician is standing behind the patient, assisting in the medial rotation of the arm. They ask the patient to 'try and hold your arm in this position'. The clinician then releases the arm (Fig. 2.5).

FINDINGS

Positive result: The patient is unable to hold the position and the arm slaps the lower back (Fig. 2.6). This may suggest the patient has a rupture or partial tear of subscapularis, or pain inhibition. A slow loss of the position may suggest a weakness in subscapularis control or pain inhibition.

Negative result: There is normal function/strength, compared to the asymptomatic side.

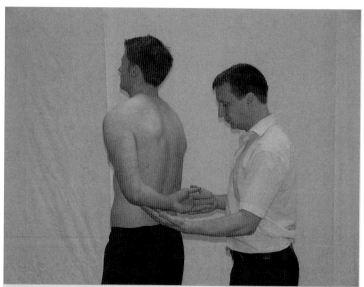

Fig 2.5 Lift off test. The clinician assists the patient into full shoulder medial rotation so that the hand is not touching the small of the back and asks the patient to hold this position.

Table 2.3 Sensitivity and specificity values of the lift off test

Author	Aim of study	Design	Sensitivity	Specificity
Leroux et al (1995)	To assess the diagnostic value of clinical tests for shoulder impingement syndrome	Correlation of 55 subjects' preoperative test findings with surgery findings	0%	61%

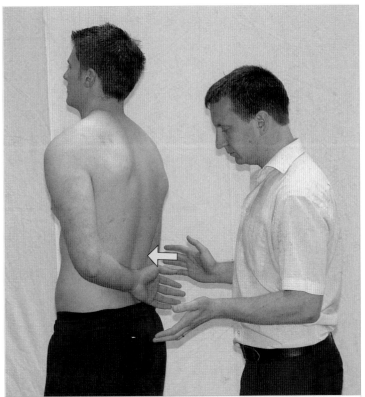

Fig 2.6   Lift off test. A positive result; the hand falls towards the patient's back.

HORNBLOWER'S TEST

Hornblower's test is designed to test the integrity of the posterior aspect of the rotator cuff, in particular the teres minor muscle. The procedure of the test involves asking the patient to bring their hands to their mouth without their shoulder abducting to 90°. The ability to bring their hand to their mouth needs a stabilizing action of lateral rotation from teres minor. Without this action the patient uses shoulder abduction to hold their hand to their mouth, as if blowing a horn. An expected positive response is the inability of the patient to adopt the hand to mouth position without abducting the shoulder joint.

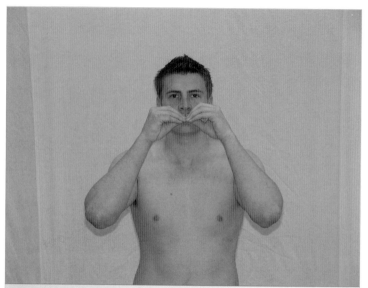

Fig 2.7 Hornblower's test. The patient is able to bring both hands to their mouth without needing to abduct the shoulder.

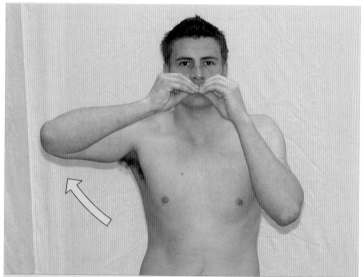

Fig 2.8 Hornblower's test. The patient's right shoulder has abducted, suggesting possible weakness.

PROCEDURE

Patient: The patient is positioned in sitting or standing. The clinician asks the patient to bring their hand to their mouth while keeping their shoulders in a neutral position (Fig. 2.7).

Clinician: The clinician is standing in front of the patient, assessing the ability and quality of the movement. The clinician can ask the patient to perform this test bilaterally so that a comparison can be made between the affected and the non-affected side.

FINDINGS

Positive result: The patient lifts their hand to their mouth but abducts their shoulder to approximately 90° to do so (Fig. 2.8). Active abduction of the shoulder may suggest a complete or partial tear of teres minor or another aspect of the posterior rotator cuff.

Negative result: The patient is able to adopt the position requested equal to the non-affected side.

Table 2.4 Sensitivity and specificity values of Hornblower's test

Author	Aim of study	Design	Sensitivity	Specificity
Walch et al (1998)	To correlate the 'dropping' and 'Hornblower's' sign with fatty degeneration of teres minor identified using CT arthrogram	Correlation of 54 subjects' clinical test findings with CT arthrogram findings	100%	93%

NEER'S IMPINGEMENT TEST

Neer's impingement test is designed to test for impingement of the shoulder; it may also aid in the identification of rotator cuff disease/pathology. The procedure of the test involves placing the shoulder joint into flexion and medial rotation. The clinician then passively flexes the shoulder; this action decreases the available subacromial space and potentially 'impinges' soft tissue structures between the anterior margin of the acromion and the head of the humerus or the superior aspect of the glenoid. An expected positive response from this test is to reproduce the patient's pain.

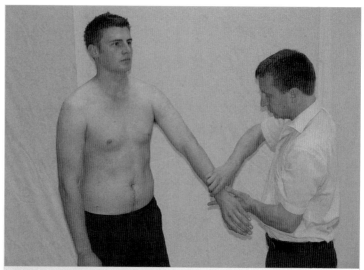

Fig 2.9   Neer's impingement test. The clinician assists the patient in slight flexion and medial rotation.

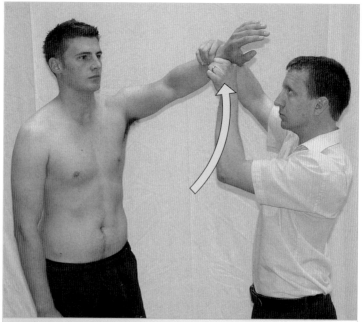

Fig 2.10   Neer's impingement test. The patient's arm is assisted through flexion.

PROCEDURE

Patient: The patient is positioned in standing. Their shoulder is flexed to 20° and fully medially rotated (Fig. 2.9).

Clinician: The clinician is standing in front of the patient, assisting the movement of the patient's arm through shoulder flexion (Fig. 2.10).

FINDINGS

Positive result: Pain reported by the patient on the antero-lateral aspect of the shoulder between 80° and 140° of shoulder flexion may suggest impingement of the shoulder.

Negative result: There is no reproduction of pain during the test procedure.

Table 2.5 Sensitivity and specificity values of Neer's impingement test

Author	Aim of study	Design	Sensitivity	Specificity
Calis et al (2000)	To investigate the diagnostic values of clinical diagnostic tests in subacromial impingement syndrome	Correlation of 120 subjects' preoperative test findings with MRI findings	88.7%	30.5%
Leroux et al (1995)	To determine the diagnostic value of clinical tests for shoulder impingement	Correlation of 55 subjects' preoperative test findings with open surgery and arthroscopy	89%	Not reported
Park et al (2005)	To determine the diagnostic accuracy of clinical tests for the different degrees of subacromial impingement syndrome	Correlation of 552 subjects' preoperative test findings with arthroscopic findings	68.0%	68.7%

HAWKINS–KENNEDY IMPINGEMENT TEST

The Hawkins–Kennedy impingement test is designed to test for impingement of the shoulder; it may also aid in the identification of rotator cuff disease/pathology. The procedure of the test involves placing the shoulder joint into a position of flexion and medial rotation. This position is thought to increase the 'impingement' of the subacromial space by the clinician providing an increased medial rotational force to push the head of the humerus or the superior aspect of the glenoid up against the acromion, in turn, impinging the soft tissue structures. An expected positive response from this test is to reproduce the patient's pain.

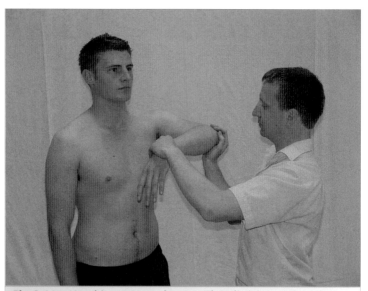

Fig 2.11   Hawkins–Kennedy test. The clinician assists the patient's shoulder into 90° flexion and medial rotation.

PROCEDURE

Patient: The patient is positioned in standing. Their shoulder is flexed to 90° in full medial rotation and their elbow is in 90° of flexion (Fig. 2.11).

Clinician: The clinician is standing in front of the patient, supporting the limb to be tested, and pushing downwards on the patient's wrist. The clinician applies medial rotation to the arm, through the full available range (Fig. 2.12).

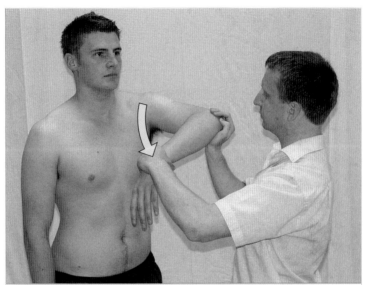

Fig 2.12 Hawkins–Kennedy test. The clinician applies a downwards pressure to the patient's wrist, increasing medial rotation of the shoulder.

FINDINGS

Positive result: Pain reported by the patient on the antero-lateral aspect of the shoulder which intensifies with increased application of medial rotation may suggest impingement of the shoulder.

Negative result: There is no reproduction of pain during the test procedure.

Table 2.6 Sensitivity and specificity values of the Hawkins–Kennedy impingement test

Author	Aim of study	Design	Sensitivity	Specificity
Calis et al (2000)	To investigate the diagnostic values of clinical diagnostic tests in subacromial impingement syndrome	Correlation of 120 subjects' preoperative test findings with MRI findings	92.1%	25.0%

(table continues)

Table 2.6 (continued)

Author	Aim of study	Design	Sensitivity	Specificity
Leroux et al (1995)	To determine the diagnostic value of clinical tests for shoulder impingement	Correlation of 55 subjects' preoperative test findings with open surgery and arthroscopy	87%	Not reported
Park et al (2005)	To determine the diagnostic accuracy of clinical tests for the different degrees of subacromial impingement syndrome	Correlation of 552 subjects' preoperative test findings with arthroscopic findings	71.5%	66.3%

YOCUM'S TEST

Yocum's test is designed to test for impingement of the shoulder; it may also aid in the identification of rotator cuff disease/pathology. The procedure of the test involves positioning the patient's hand on to their opposite shoulder and lifting the elbow. This position may impinge soft tissue structures within the anterior aspect of the subacromial space between the tuberosities of the head of the humerus and the acromion process. An expected positive response from this test is to reproduce the patient's pain.

PROCEDURE
Patient: The patient is positioned in standing or sitting. The hand of the upper limb to be tested is placed on the opposite shoulder (Fig. 2.13).
Clinician: The clinician is positioned in front or to the side of the patient, to assist in the raising of the elbow, as far as it will go. The clinician should also stabilize the patient's scapula (Fig. 2.14).

FINDINGS
Positive result: Pain reported by the patient around the subacromial space area of the shoulder may suggest signs of impingement or potential rotator cuff pathology.
Negative result: There is no reproduction of pain during test procedure.

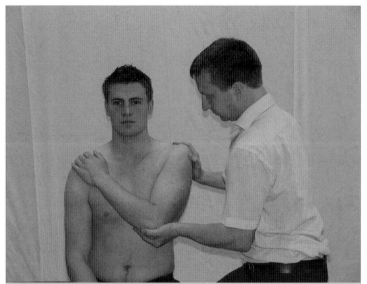

Fig 2.13 Yocum's test. The clinician assists the patient's hand to the opposite shoulder.

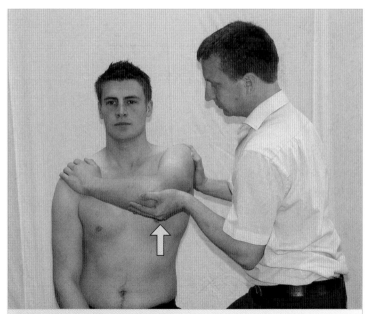

Fig 2.14 Yocum's test. The clinician passively raises the patient's elbow while stabilizing their scapula.

Table 2.7 Sensitivity and specificity values of Yocum's test

Author	Aim of study	Design	Sensitivity	Specificity
Leroux et al (1995)	To assess the diagnostic value of clinical tests for shoulder impingement syndrome	Correlation of 55 subjects' preoperative test findings with open surgery and arthroscopy	78%	Not reported

PAINFUL ARC TEST

The painful arc test is designed to test for impingement of the shoulder; it may also aid in the identification of rotator cuff disease/pathology. The procedure of the test involves active abduction of the upper limb. As abduction takes place the subacromial space, between the tuberosities of the humerus and the acromion, is reduced maximally between 60° and 120° of movement. Between these ranges the bony structures may impinge on any soft tissue structure in the subacromial space and thus cause pain in the mid-range of abduction. An expected positive response from this test is to reproduce the patient's pain and/or demonstrate muscle weakness.

PROCEDURE

Patient: The patient is positioned in standing. On the clinician's command they raise the affected limb slowly through abduction from 0° to 180°, or as far as possible (Figs 2.15 and 2.16).
Clinician: The clinician is standing in front or behind the patient, to assess the quality of movement. The patient is asked to report the onset and remission of pain during the movement.

FINDINGS

Positive result: Pain reported by the patient between 60° and 120° of abduction. Pain often decreases after 120° of abduction. A failure to achieve the movement due to pain may indicate pain inhibition. A failure to achieve the movement due to weakness (+/− pain) may indicate muscle weakness or a muscle tear.
Negative result: There is no pain reported and there is normal function.

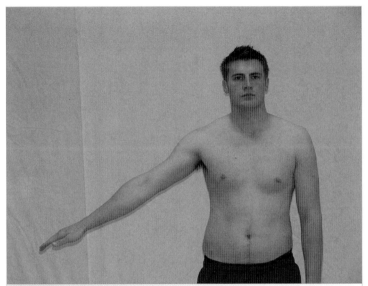

Fig 2.15 Painful arc test. The patient is asked to abduct their arm as far as it will go.

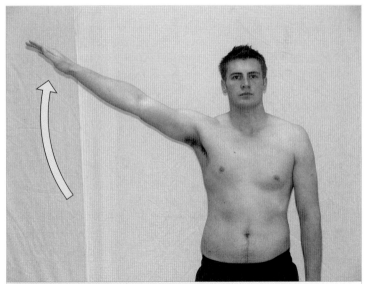

Fig 2.16 Painful arc test. A positive result; pain reported between 60° and 120° abduction.

Table 2.8 Sensitivity and specificity values of the painful arc test

Author	Aim of study	Design	Sensitivity	Specificity
Calis et al (2000)	To investigate the diagnostic values of clinical diagnostic tests in subacromial impingement syndrome	Correlation of 120 subjects' preoperative test findings with MRI findings	32.5%	80.5%
Park et al (2005)	To determine the diagnostic accuracy of clinical tests for the different degrees of subacromial impingement syndrome	Correlation of 552 subjects' preoperative test findings with arthroscopic findings	73.5%	81.1%

DROP ARM TEST

The drop arm test is designed to test for impingement of the shoulder; it may also aid in the identification of rotator cuff disease/pathology. The procedure of the test involves the patient slowly lowering their arm from an abducted shoulder position. As adduction occurs, deltoid relinquishes its control of the movement and the rotator cuff muscles take a more active role towards the inner range of movement. This can result in an element of control of adduction, then a sudden drop of the limb. During the movement the subacromial space may also be decreased, thus presenting signs of impingement. An expected positive response from this test is to demonstrate muscle weakness and/or reproduce the patient's pain.

PROCEDURE
Patient: The patient is positioned in standing or sitting. Their shoulder is positioned into greater than 90° of abduction.
Clinician: The clinician is standing behind the subject, ready to support the tested limb as required. The patient is asked to slowly lower their arm back to their side (Fig. 2.17).

FINDINGS
Positive result: The arm drops to the patient's side, with or without the report of pain; this may suggest a complete or partial rotator cuff tear or signs of impingement. The patient lowers their

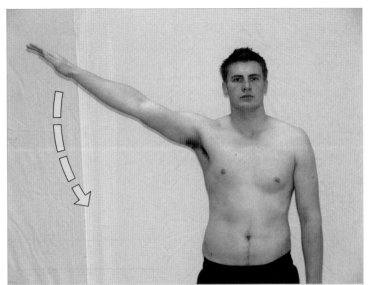

Fig 2.17   Drop arm test. The patient slowly lowers their arm from an abducted position.

arm slowly to their side but has poor control over the movement; this may suggest a partial tear or weakness in the rotator cuff muscles. This may also indicate pain inhibition.

Negative result: There is no pain reported, normal function/ strength and a smooth lowering of limb, similar to the asymptomatic side.

Table 2.9 Sensitivity and specificity values of the drop arm test

Author	Aim of study	Design	Sensitivity	Specificity
Calis et al (2000)	To investigate the diagnostic values of clinical diagnostic tests in subacromial impingement syndrome	Correlation of 120 subjects' preoperative test findings with MRI findings	7.8%	97.2%
Park et al (2005)	To determine the diagnostic accuracy of clinical tests for the different degrees of subacromial impingement syndrome	Correlation of 552 subjects' preoperative test findings with arthroscopic findings	26.9%	88.4%

APPREHENSION TEST

The apprehension test is designed to test for anterior instability of the glenohumeral joint. The procedure of the test involves positioning the shoulder into abduction and full lateral rotation. As the name of the test suggests, this position is designed to give the patient a feeling of apprehension, as if the shoulder could be vulnerable to dislocation. With this in mind, caution should be paramount when applying this test as there is potential risk of further dislocation of the shoulder. An expected positive response from this test is reluctance by the patient to adopt this position, because of the feeling of instability.

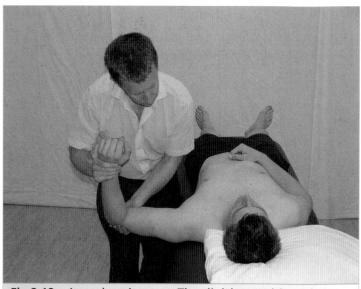

Fig 2.18 Apprehension test. The clinician positions the patient into 90° abduction while supporting the elbow.

PROCEDURE

Patient: The patient is positioned in supine on a plinth. Their shoulder is abducted to 90° and their elbow flexed to 90° (Fig. 2.18).

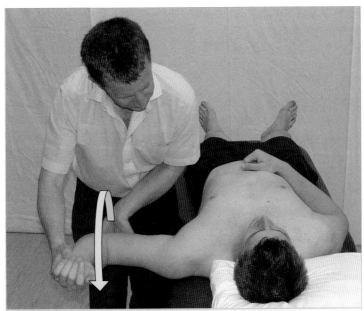

Fig 2.19 Apprehension test. The clinician slowly applies lateral rotation and monitors the patient for signs of apprehension.

Clinician: The patient is informed of the test procedure and reminded to report symptoms of 'apprehension'. The clinician is positioned standing alongside the patient, supporting the upper limb, and applies up to 90° lateral rotation of the humerus (Fig. 2.19). The clinician stops immediately if the patient reports apprehension or even looks apprehensive during the movement.

FINDINGS

Positive result: As lateral rotation is applied from 0° towards 90° the patient reports a feeling of instability, apprehension, vulnerability or pain during movement. This may indicate an element of anterior instability of the glenohumeral joint.

Negative result: As the clinician fully laterally rotates the arm, no apprehension is reported by the patient.

Table 2.10 Sensitivity and specificity values of the apprehension test

Author	Aim of study	Design	Sensitivity	Specificity
Farber et al (2006)	To determine the clinical value of the apprehension, relocation and anterior drawer tests for the diagnosis of traumatic anterior shoulder instability	Correlation of 46 subjects' clinical test findings with arthroscopy findings	For pain 50% For apprehension 72%	For pain 56% For apprehension 96%
Guanche & Jones (2003)	An evaluation of seven clinical tests for tears of the glenoid labrum	Correlation of 61 subjects' clinical test findings with arthroscopy findings	For any labral tear 40% For SLAP lesion only 30%	For any labral tear 87% For SLAP lesion only 63%
Lo et al (2004)	To assess the validity of the apprehension, relocation and surprise tests as predictors of anterior shoulder instability	Correlation of 46 subjects' clinical test findings with diagnostic categories	52.78%	98.91%

APPREHENSION RELOCATION TEST

The apprehension relocation test is designed to test for anterior instability of the glenohumeral joint. This test is also known as 'Fowler's test'. The procedure of the test follows the same principle and positioning as the apprehension test; however, when the patient is at the point of apprehension, the clinician applies a posteriorly directed force to the humeral head, thus 'reducing' or 'supporting' the instability and correspondingly reducing the feeling of apprehension. With this in mind, caution should be paramount when applying this test because of the potential risk of further dislocation of the shoulder. An expected positive response from this test is a reduction of the patient's feeling of apprehension as the posterior force is applied to the glenohumeral joint.

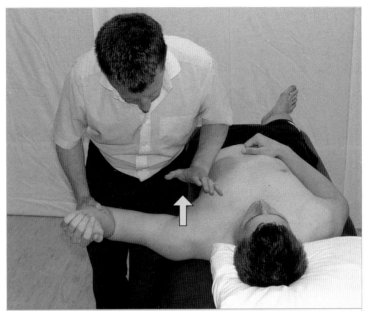

Fig 2.20 Apprehension relocation test. The clinician slowly applies lateral rotation until the patient reports apprehension.

PROCEDURE

Patient: The patient is positioned in supine on a plinth. Their shoulder abducted to 90° and their elbow flexed to 90°.

Clinician: The patient is informed of the test procedure and reminded to report symptoms of 'apprehension'. The clinician, who is positioned standing alongside the patient, supporting the upper limb, applies up to 90° lateral rotation of the humerus (Fig. 2.20). The clinician stops immediately if the patient reports apprehension or even looks apprehensive during the movement. At this point the clinician applies an anterior to posterior force down through the head of the humerus and asks the patient if the feeling of apprehension has reduced (Fig. 2.21).

FINDINGS

Positive result: A reduction in the patient's reported feelings of apprehension suggests that the anterior to posterior force has reduced an element of instability, thus confirming potential anterior instability of the glenohumeral joint.

Negative result: As the clinician fully laterally rotates the arm, no apprehension is reported by patient and no change with the anterior to posterior force.

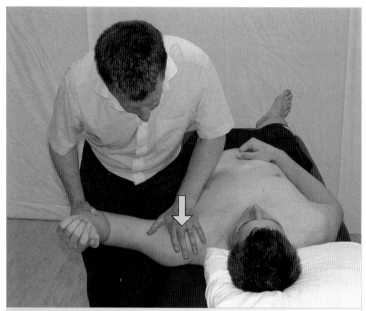

Fig 2.21 Apprehension relocation test. At the point of apprehension the clinician applies an anterior to posterior pressure to the anterior aspect of the shoulder to assess if the reported apprehension reduces.

Table 2.11 Sensitivity and specificity values of the apprehension relocation test

Author	Aim of study	Design	Sensitivity	Specificity
Farber et al (2006)	To determine the clinical value of the apprehension, relocation and anterior drawer tests for the diagnosis of traumatic anterior shoulder instability	Correlation of 46 subjects' clinical test findings with arthroscopy findings	For relief of pain 30% For relief of apprehension 81%	For relief of pain 90% For relief of apprehension 92%
Lo et al (2004)	To assess the validity of the apprehension, relocation and surprise tests as predictors of anterior shoulder instability	Correlation of 46 subjects' clinical test findings with diagnostic categories	45.83%	54.35%

APPREHENSION TEST ANTERIOR RELEASE METHOD

The apprehension test anterior release method is designed to test for anterior instability of the glenohumeral joint. This test is also known as the 'surprise method'. The procedure of the test follows the same principle and positioning as the apprehension test; however, the clinician applies the posteriorly directed force to the glenohumeral joint before lateral rotation is added to the movement combination. After the anterior to posterior force has been applied, the clinician adds the final movement of lateral rotation. The clinician then slowly releases the pressure on the anterior aspect of the joint and monitors for signs of apprehension. This technique allows for more control over the patient's apprehension symptoms and allows the clinician to reapply the pressure to reduce the feeling of apprehension as required. With this in mind, caution should be paramount when applying this test because of the potential risk of further dislocation of the shoulder. An expected positive response from this test is a feeling of apprehension as the anterior to posterior force is slowly released from the glenohumeral joint.

PROCEDURE

Patient: The patient is positioned in supine on a plinth. Their shoulder is abducted to 90° and their elbow flexed to 90°.

Clinician: The patient is informed of the test procedure and reminded to report symptoms of apprehension. The clinician is positioned alongside the patient, supporting the upper limb, while simultaneously applying an anterior to posterior pressure to the anterior aspect of the shoulder. The clinician then applies a further movement of lateral rotation, at this point, with the anterior to posterior directed pressure remaining constant (Fig. 2.22). At the end of the available range of lateral rotation, the clinician gently releases the pressure and monitors the patient for any signs of apprehension (Fig. 2.23).

FINDINGS

Positive result: As the anterior to posterior pressure applied onto the head of the humerus is released, the patient may report a feeling of instability, apprehension, vulnerability or pain. This may indicate an element of anterior instability of the glenohumeral joint.

Negative result: There is no onset of apprehension on reduction of the anterior to posterior pressure.

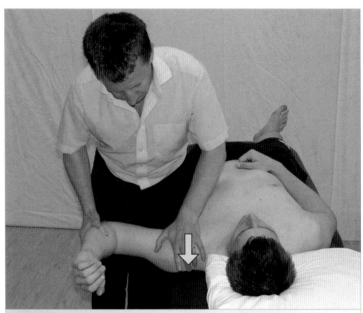

Fig 2.22 Apprehension test anterior release method. The clinician slowly applies lateral rotation while maintaining an anterior to posterior pressure to the anterior aspect of the shoulder.

Notes

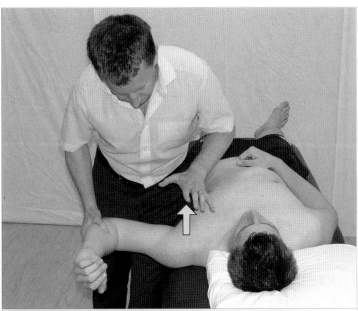

Fig 2.23 Apprehension test anterior release method. If no apprehension is reported the clinician slowly releases their hand supporting the shoulder and assesses for any further signs of apprehension.

Table 2.12 Sensitivity and specificity values of the apprehension test anterior release method

Author	Aim of study	Design	Sensitivity	Specificity
Gross & Distefano (1997)	To assess the accuracy of the anterior release test	Correlation of 37 subjects' clinical test findings with operative findings	91.9%	88.9%
Lo et al (2004)	To assess the validity of the apprehension, relocation and surprise tests as predictors of anterior shoulder instability	Correlation of 46 subjects' clinical test findings with diagnostic categories	63.89%	98.91%

APPREHENSION TEST FULCRUM METHOD

The apprehension test fulcrum method is designed to test for anterior instability of the glenohumeral joint. This test is also known as the 'augmentation method'. The procedure of the test follows the same principle and positioning as the apprehension test; however, the clinician's hand is placed under the patient's glenohumeral joint to act as a fulcrum. The act of using the hand as a fulcrum increases the scope for movement into an apprehension position. This test may be useful with patients where there is a difficulty in locating symptoms. With this in mind, caution should be paramount when applying the test because of the potential risk of further dislocation of the shoulder. An expected positive response from this test is reluctance by the patient to adopt this position, because of feelings of instability.

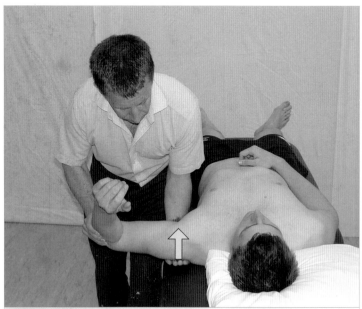

Fig 2.24 Apprehension test fulcrum method. The clinician places their hand underneath the patient's shoulder to act as a fulcrum.

PROCEDURE

Patient: The patient is positioned in supine on a plinth. Their shoulder is abducted to 90° and their elbow flexed to 90°.

Clinician: The patient is informed of the test procedure and reminded to report symptoms of apprehension. The clinician is positioned alongside the patient, supporting the upper limb while simultaneously positioning their other hand underneath the patient's shoulder joint (Fig. 2.24). This provides a fulcrum from which there is more range to move the glenohumeral joint into a vulnerable position. The clinician applies a further movement of lateral rotation and monitors for signs of apprehension (Fig. 2.25).

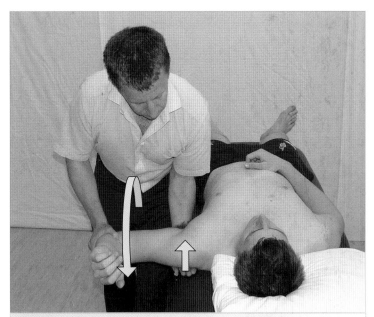

Fig 2.25 Apprehension test fulcrum method. In this position the clinician slowly applies lateral rotation and monitors the patient for signs of apprehension.

FINDINGS

Positive result: As lateral rotation increases from 0° towards 90°, a reported feeling of instability, apprehension, vulnerability or pain may suggest anterior instability of the glenohumeral joint.

Negative result: The clinician laterally rotates their arm to the maximum and no apprehension is reported by the patient.

LOAD AND SHIFT TEST

The load and shift test is designed to test for anterior instability of the glenohumeral joint. The procedure of the test involves fixing the scapula aspect of the glenohumeral joint and applying a quick yet firm anterior translation of the humeral head. The amount of anterior translation available during the movement may signify the amount of instability present in the joint. If a previous subluxation or dislocation has taken place the soft tissue structures that support the joint are more lax than normal and thus allow anterior translation to take place. An expected positive result of this test is an increased degree of anterior translation of the humeral head on the glenoid of the scapula.

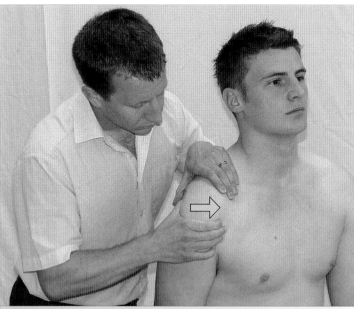

Fig 2.26 Load and shift test. The clinician fixes the scapula with one hand and applies an anterior translation force to the humeral head with the other.

PROCEDURE

Patient: The patient is positioned in sitting, their arm relaxed by their side, with their forearm supported if required.

Clinician: The clinician stands behind the patient. They have one hand positioned over the patient's shoulder, fixing the scapula.

Their other hand provides a firm grip on the humeral head. The hand gripping the humeral head then applies an anterior translation of the humeral head (Fig. 2.26).

FINDINGS
  Possible findings: The Hawkins and Bokor classification system provides a framework to establish the severity of the laxity of the shoulder for anterior subluxation and dislocation (Tzannes & Murrell 2002).

  Grade 1 = Translation of the humeral head to the glenoid rim, but not over it. (The clinician may feel a slight pulling out of the humeral head as it rides against the lip of the glenoid.)
  Grade 2 = Translation of the humeral head over the glenoid rim, but immediately and spontaneously reduces back to its normal position. (The clinician feels the movement of the humeral head over the rim of the glenoid and may feel the relocation of the head.)
  Grade 3 = The humeral head dislocates from the glenoid fossa and does not return to its original location when the clinician removes their translating hand from the humeral head.

MODIFIED ANTERIOR DRAWER TEST

The modified anterior drawer test is designed to test for anterior shoulder instability. The procedure of the test involves fixing the scapular aspect of the glenohumeral joint and applying a slow and firm anterior translation of the humeral head while the shoulder is positioned in 60–80° of abduction. The amount of anterior translation available during the movement may signify the amount of instability present in the joint. If a previous subluxation or dislocation has taken place the soft tissue structures that support the joint are more lax than normal, and thus allow the anterior translation to take place. An expected positive result of this test is an increased degree of anterior translation of the humeral head on the glenoid of the scapula.

PROCEDURE
  Patient: The patient is positioned in supine on a plinth. Their shoulder is abducted to between 60° and 80° with 0° of shoulder rotation and their elbow in 90° of flexion.
  Clinician: The clinician is standing to the side of the plinth, taking the full weight of the limb to ensure the patient is relaxed

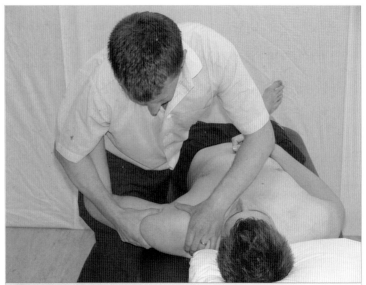

Fig 2.27 Modified anterior drawer test. The clinician fixes the scapula with one hand and grasps the humeral head with the other.

(Fig. 2.27). This will allow minimal muscle activity to allow free movement of the humeral head. The clinician then grasps the humeral head and translates it anteriorly (Fig. 2.28).

FINDINGS

Possible findings: The Hawkins and Bokor classification system provides a framework to establish the severity of the laxity of the shoulder for anterior subluxation and dislocation (Tzannes & Murrell 2002).

Grade 1 = Translation of the humeral head to the glenoid rim, but not over it. (The clinician may feel a slight pulling out of the humeral head as it rides against the lip of the glenoid.)

Grade 2 = Translation of the humeral head over the glenoid rim, but immediately and spontaneously reduces back to its normal position. (The clinician feels the movement of the humeral head over the rim of the glenoid and may feel the relocation of the head.)

Grade 3 = The humeral head dislocates from the glenoid fossa and does not return to its original location when the clinician removes their translating hand from the humeral head.

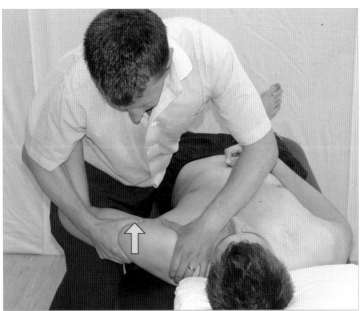

Fig 2.28 Modified anterior drawer test. The clinician draws the humeral head anteriorly and assesses for signs of instability.

Table 2.13 Sensitivity and specificity values of the modified anterior drawer test

Author	Aim of study	Design	Sensitivity	Specificity
Farber et al (2006)	To determine the clinical value of the apprehension, relocation and anterior drawer tests for the diagnosis of traumatic anterior shoulder instability	Correlation of 46 subjects' clinical test findings with arthroscopy findings	For pain 28% For reproduction of symptoms 53%	For pain 71% For reproduction of symptoms 85%

POSTERIOR DRAWER TEST

The posterior drawer test is designed to test for posterior instability of the glenohumeral joint. The procedure of the test involves positioning the joint in an abducted, flexed and medially rotated position. The clinician applies a posterior force to the joint through the length of the humerus. This force attempts to recreate the position of instability by pushing the head of the humerus out of the posterior aspect of the shoulder joint. The clinician may change the position of the shoulder joint to 'explore' the point of instability. An expected positive response from this test is an increased degree of posterior translation of the humeral head on the glenoid of the scapula.

PROCEDURE
Patient: The patient is positioned in supine on a plinth. The shoulder is positioned in 100–120° of abduction and slight flexion. The elbow is positioned in 120° of flexion.
Clinician: The clinician is standing alongside the patient. One hand supports the patient's scapula by grasping over the top of the shoulder. The other hand takes a firm hold of the elbow (Fig. 2.29). The clinician applies a medial rotation movement and a posterior force to the shoulder joint, transmitted along the length of the humerus. The clinician can then alter the degree of abduction, flexion or medial rotation to try and identify the position of instability (Fig. 2.30).

FINDINGS
Positive result: Increased range of posterior translation of the affected limb with either evidence of subluxation or, less frequently, dislocation of the humeral head may suggest posterior instability of the glenohumeral joint. The test may also reproduce the patient's symptoms.
Negative result: There is no obvious increase in the range of translation from the affected side to the non-affected side and no reproduction of their symptoms.

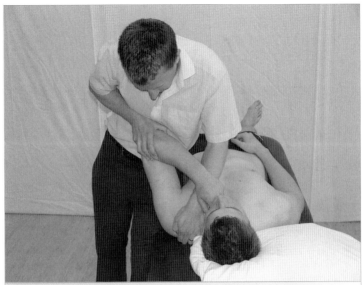

Fig 2.29   Posterior drawer test. The clinician stabilizes the scapula while maintaining the abducted and medially rotated position of the glenohumeral joint.

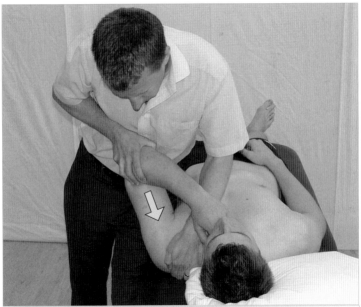

Fig 2.30   Posterior drawer test. The clinician applies a force down through the humeral shaft and assesses for signs of instability.

POSTERIOR SUBLUXATION TEST

The posterior subluxation test is designed to test for posterior instability of the glenohumeral joint. This test is also known as the 'jerk test'. The procedure of the test involves positioning the joint into an adducted, flexed and medially rotated position. The clinician applies a posterior force to the joint through the length of the humerus. This force attempts to recreate the position of instability by pushing the head of the humerus out of the posterior aspect of the shoulder joint. An expected positive response from this test is an increased degree of posterior translation of the humeral head on the glenoid of the scapula. A 'jerk' or 'click' may also be evident as the humeral head moves posteriorly on the glenoid.

PROCEDURE

Patient: The patient is positioned in supine on a plinth. Their shoulder joint is positioned in 90° of flexion, slight adduction and medial rotation.

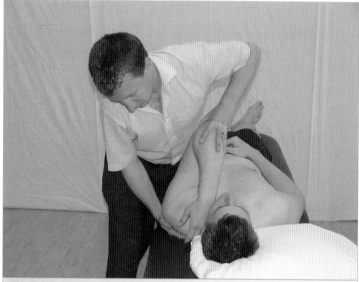

Fig 2.31   Posterior subluxation test. The clinician positions one hand on the posterior aspect of the joint line to palpate for signs of instability.

Clinician: The clinician is standing by the patient. They have one hand applying a force down through the shaft of the humerus via the elbow. The other hand is placed on the posterior joint line

(Fig. 2.31). The clinician applies an anterior to posterior force through the shoulder joint (Fig. 2.32).

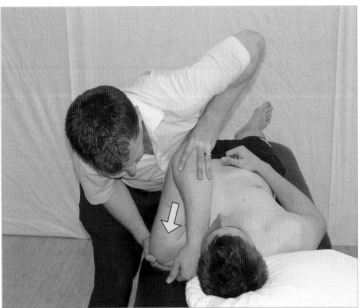

Fig 2.32   Posterior subluxation test. The clinician applies a force through the shaft of the humerus and assesses for signs of instability.

Table 2.14 Sensitivity and specificity values of the posterior subluxation test

Author	Aim of study	Design	Sensitivity	Specificity
Kim et al (2005)	To evaluate the presence or absence of pain with the jerk test as a predictor of the success of nonoperative treatment for posteroinferior instability of the shoulder and to identify the pathological lesion responsible for the pain in the jerk test	Correlation of 172 shoulders' clinical test findings with arthroscopic findings	73%	98%

FINDINGS

Positive result: A sudden 'jerk' or 'click' with a palpable feeling of posterior movement of the humeral head may suggest a posterior instability of the glenohumeral joint.

Negative result: There is no obvious increase in range of translation from affected side to non-affected side and no reproduction of their symptoms.

SULCUS SIGN

The sulcus sign refers to the observation of the skin and soft tissue around the shoulder joint. An abnormal dip or 'sulcus' identified on the lateral aspect of the shoulder over the subacromial space may suggest inferior instability of the glenohumeral joint. As a result of the lack of muscle or soft tissue control around the shoulder the humerus often hangs lower than normal and thus creates a dip in the subacromial space, under the acromion. The clinician may exacerbate this further by applying a gradual downwards distraction force to the glenohumeral joint. An expected positive finding of this test is the observation of a dip under the acromion on the lateral aspect of the shoulder.

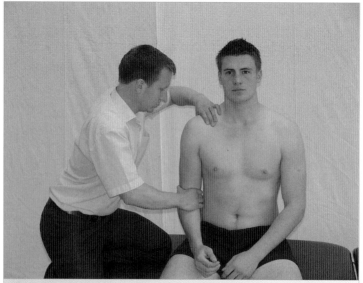

Fig 2.33 Sulcus sign. The clinician stabilizes the scapula and grasps the elbow proximal to the joint line.

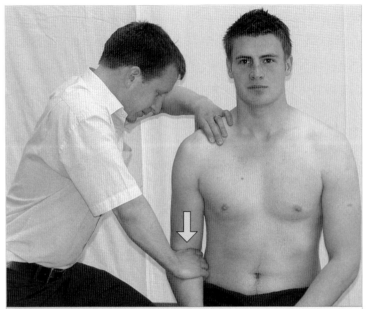

Fig 2.34 Sulcus sign. The clinician applies a downwards force attempting to drag the humeral head inferiorly on the glenoid fossa.

PROCEDURE

Patient: The patient is positioned in sitting, with their arm relaxed by their side.

Clinician: The clinician stands or sits by the side of the patient, grasps their arm at the elbow with one hand and stabilizes the scapula with the other (Fig. 2.33). A gradual inferior pull is applied to the humerus, attempting to pull the humeral head down on the glenoid fossa (Fig. 2.34).

FINDINGS

Positive result: Identification of a subacromial sulcus on the affected limb may suggest inferior instability of the glenohumeral joint.

Negative result: There is no identification of a subacromial sulcus on the affected limb.

CLUNK TEST

The clunk test is designed to test for a labral tear of the glenoid labrum within the glenohumeral joint. The procedure of the test involves an anterior movement of the humeral head against the glenoid in a fully abducted shoulder position. The translation of the humeral head acts to 'catch' the torn piece of the labrum. This is perceived as a 'click' or a 'catch' as the humeral head moves over the affected piece of the labrum. An expected positive response from this test is an audible and/or palpable click or catch within the shoulder joint.

PROCEDURE

Patient: The patient is positioned in supine on a plinth. Their shoulder is abducted fully, and laterally rotated.

Clinician: The clinician stands on the side of patient to be tested, supporting the limb with their opposite arm. The clinician applies an anteriorly directed force from the posterior aspect of the glenohumeral joint with one hand (Fig. 2.35) and maintains lateral rotation with the other. The clinician pushes through the shaft of the humerus, while maintaining lateral rotation (Fig. 2.36).

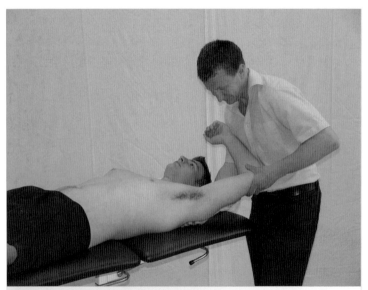

Fig 2.35   Clunk test. The clinician applies an anteriorly directed force with one hand under the shoulder.

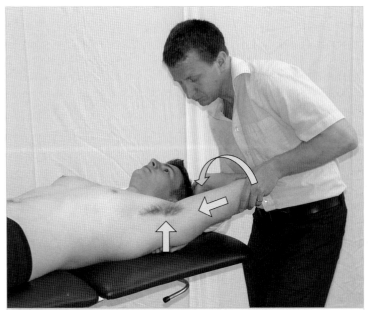

Fig 2.36 Clunk test. The clinician then applies lateral rotation and compression through the shaft of the humerus and assesses for a deep 'click' or 'catch' during the movement.

FINDINGS

Positive result: A deep 'click' or 'catch' perceived by the patient may be indicative of the humeral head catching the labrum and, hence, may suggest a tear of the glenoid labrum.

Negative result: There is no deep 'click' or 'catch' felt on application of the test.

CRANK TEST

The crank test is designed to test for a tear of the glenoid labrum within the glenohumeral joint. The procedure of the test involves a rotational movement of the humeral head against the glenoid in an abducted shoulder position while the clinician applies a force through the shaft of the humerus to compress the joint. The rotation and compression force acts to 'catch' the torn piece of the labrum. This is perceived as a 'click', 'clunk' or 'catch' as the humeral head moves over the affected piece of the labrum.

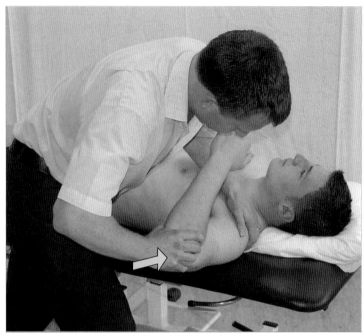

Fig 2.37 Crank test. The clinician stabilizes the scapula with one hand and applies a force down through the shaft of the humerus.

An expected positive response from this test is reproduction of the patient's pain with or without an audible or palpable click within the shoulder joint.

PROCEDURE
Patient: The patient is positioned in sitting or supine on a plinth. Their shoulder is abducted to 90° and the elbow flexed to 120°.
Clinician: The clinician is standing to the side of the patient, supporting their shoulder with one hand and gripping the elbow with the other. The hand on the elbow transmits a force through the axis of the humerus (Fig. 2.37). When the compression force is applied, the clinician laterally and medially rotates the shoulder (Fig. 2.38).

FINDINGS
Positive result: Reproduction of the patient's pain, with or without an audible or palpable 'click' within the shoulder joint,

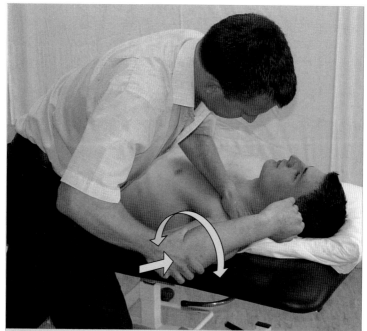

Fig 2.38 Crank test. The clinician then applies medial and lateral rotation and assesses for a deep 'click' within the shoulder joint.

may be indicative of the humeral head catching part of the labrum and, hence, may suggest a tear of the glenoid labrum.
Negative result: There is no reported catching or reproduction of symptoms.

O'BRIEN'S TEST

O'Brien's test is designed to test for a labral tear of the glenoid labrum within the glenohumeral joint. This test is also known as the 'active compression test'. The procedure of the test involves using the upper limb as a lever to apply force on to the long head of biceps and, in turn, the superior labrum. Loading a flexed shoulder with an internally rotated upper limb pulls on the long head of biceps and the superior aspect of the glenoid labrum. An expected positive result from this test is the reproduction of the patient's pain.

PROCEDURE

Patient: The patient is positioned in standing. The shoulder is positioned in 90° flexion, in 10° adduction, and in full medial rotation for the first part of the test and full lateral rotation for the second part of the test.

Clinician: While the shoulder is in full medial rotation the clinician stands in front of the patient, applying a downwards pressure to the distal end of the upper limb, with the patient resisting the force (Fig. 2.39). Secondly, the palm is turned upwards, laterally rotating the humerus, and the resistance is reapplied (Fig. 2.40).

FINDINGS

Positive result: In the medially rotated position pain is elicited on the anterior aspect of the shoulder, while, in the laterally rotated position, if the pain decreases it may suggest a superior labral detachment.

Negative result: There is no pain elicited on applying the test.

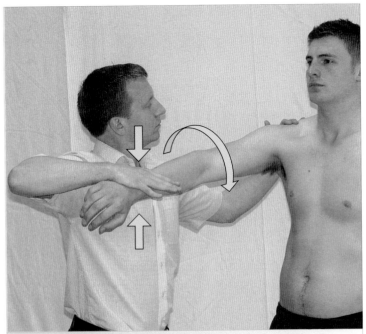

Fig 2.39 O'Brien's test. The clinician loads the patient's arm in a medially rotated position and assesses for pain.

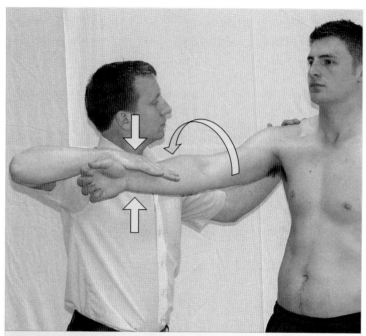

Fig 2.40   O'Brien's test. The clinician repeats the test in a laterally rotated position and assesses for pain.

Notes

Table 2.15 Sensitivity and specificity values of O'Brien's test

Author	Aim of study	Design	Sensitivity	Specificity
McFarland et al (2002)	To determine the clinical value of (three) tests commonly used during physical examination to detect SLAP lesions	Correlation of 426 subjects' clinical test findings with arthroscopic findings	47%	55%
O'Brien et al (1998)	An evaluation of the efficacy of the active compression test for diagnosing labral tears and acromioclavicular joint abnormality	Correlation of 318 subjects' clinical test findings with various combinations of radiography, MRI and clinical data	100%	95.2%
Stetson & Templin (2002)	To determine if the crank or O'Brien test was a reliable tool for detecting glenoid labrum tears	Correlation of 65 subjects' clinical test findings with arthroscopic findings	54%	31%
Walton et al (2004)	To determine the diagnostic values of tests for acromioclavicular joint pain	Correlation of 113 subjects' clinical test findings with MRI findings and bone scans	16%	90%

ANTERIOR SLIDE TEST

The anterior slide test is designed to test for a labral tear of the glenoid labrum within the glenohumeral joint. The procedure of the test involves the clinician positioning the patient's glenohumeral joint and applying a posterior to superior force to the shoulder. The force acts to move the humeral head against the labrum; if a tear is present the humeral head will catch the torn piece of labrum and elicit an audible 'click' and/or reproduce deep pain within the shoulder joint. An expected positive result from this test is an audible 'click' and/or the reproduction of the patient's pain within the shoulder joint.

PROCEDURE

Patient: The patient is positioned in sitting on a plinth. The shoulder is positioned in slight abduction with the patient's hand on their hip with their thumb facing forwards.

Clinician: The clinician is positioned behind the patient, stabilizing the scapula with one hand (Fig. 2.41). With the other hand the clinician applies a posterior to superior force from the posterior aspect of the shoulder joint (Fig. 2.42).

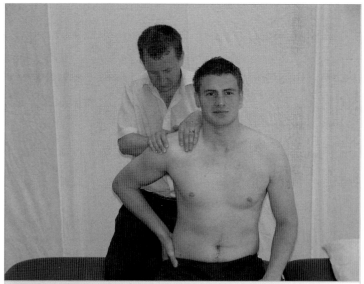

Fig 2.41   Anterior slide test. The clinician stabilizes the scapula with one hand and applies a posterior to superior force with the other.

FINDINGS

Positive result: An audible 'click' and/or deep pain reported within the shoulder joint may suggest a superior labral detachment.

Negative result: No audible 'click' and/or pain is elicited on applying the test.

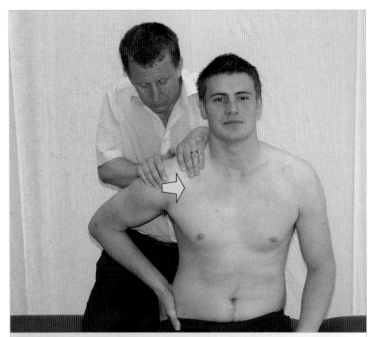

Fig 2.42 Anterior slide test. An audible 'click' or reported pain represents a positive result.

Table 2.16 Sensitivity and specificity values of the anterior slide test

Author	Aim of study	Design	Sensitivity	Specificity
McFarland et al (2002)	To determine the clinical value of (three) tests commonly used during physical examination to detect SLAP lesions	Correlation of 426 subjects' clinical test findings with arthroscopic findings	8%	84%

SPEED'S TEST

Speed's test is designed to test for a long head of biceps tendon pathology or a superior labral tear; it may also aid in the identification of impingement-type symptoms. The procedure of the test involves the clinician providing resistance to the arm as the shoulder moves from an extended position to a flexed position. This resistance is thought to load the long head of biceps tendon and thus potentially reproduce the patient's symptoms. Furthermore, the test may compress soft tissue structures within the anterior aspect of the subacromial space and thus indicate potential impingement signs. An expected positive response from this test is to reproduce the patient's pain and/or demonstrate muscle weakness.

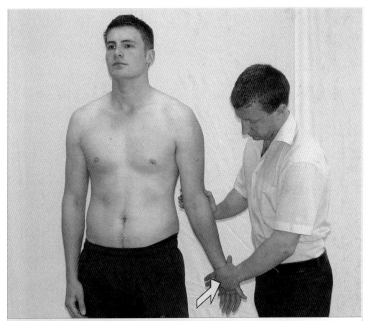

Fig 2.43 Speed's test. The patient is positioned into shoulder extension and full supination; the clinician maintains elbow extension.

PROCEDURE
Patient: The patient is positioned in standing. The shoulder is in a neutral position or slight extension, the elbow is in extension and the wrist is fully supinated (Fig. 2.43).

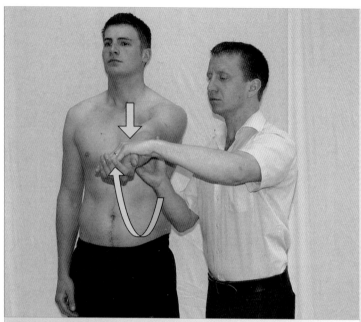

Fig 2.44 Speed's test. The patient performs shoulder flexion through to 90° as the clinician applies resistance.

Clinician: The clinician is standing to the side of the patient, applying a resistance to the distal end of the tested limb. The resistance is applied to the wrist while the patient is instructed to flex their shoulder forwards to 90° (Fig. 2.44). Equal resistance is applied throughout the procedure to allow all the movement to occur against resistance.

FINDINGS

Positive result: Reported pain located over the bicipital groove area of the humerus may indicate bicipital tendon pathology. A failure to achieve movement due to pain may indicate pain inhibition. A failure to achieve movement due to weakness (+/− pain) may indicate a muscle weakness or a rupture of the long head of biceps.

Negative result: There is no pain reported and there is normal function.

Table 2.17 Sensitivity and specificity values of Speed's test

Author	Aim of study	Design	Sensitivity	Specificity
Bennett (1998)	To determine the diagnostic accuracy of Speed's test via the arthroscopic technique for evaluating the biceps tendon	Correlation of 46 subjects' preoperative test findings with arthroscopic findings	90%	13.8%
Calis et al (2000)	To investigate the diagnostic values of clinical diagnostic tests in subacromial impingement syndrome	Correlation of 120 subjects' preoperative test findings with MRI findings	68.5%	55.5%
Guanche & Jones (2003)	An evaluation of seven clinical tests for tears of the glenoid labrum	Correlation of 61 subjects' clinical test findings with arthroscopy findings	For SLAP lesion only 9%	For SLAP lesion only 74%
Holtby & Razmjou (2004)	Explore and describe reasons for variations in diagnostic accuracy of clinical tests in predicting biceps tendon pathology and SLAP lesions	Correlation of 152 subjects' preoperative test findings with surgical findings	32%	75%
Park et al (2005)	To determine the diagnostic accuracy of clinical tests for the different degrees of subacromial impingement syndrome	Correlation of 552 subjects' preoperative test findings with arthroscopic findings	38.3%	83.3%

YERGASON'S TEST

Yergason's test is designed to test for long head of biceps tendon pathology. The procedure of the test involves resisted supination of the elbow by applying resistance at the patient's wrist. Yergason's test uses the principle of resisted supination of the elbow joint to test the proximal attachment of the long head of biceps since it is a two joint muscle. As resisted supination occurs, the force pulls on the long head of biceps within the shoulder joint. An expected positive response from this test would be reproduction of the patient's pain in the shoulder region.

PROCEDURE

Patient: The patient is positioned in standing. Their shoulder is in neutral, with the elbow in 90° flexion, and their wrist is fully pronated (Fig. 2.45).

Clinician: The clinician is standing in front of the patient, holding on to their hand. The clinician asks the patient to supinate their wrist and then applies a resistance to oppose the supination (Fig. 2.46).

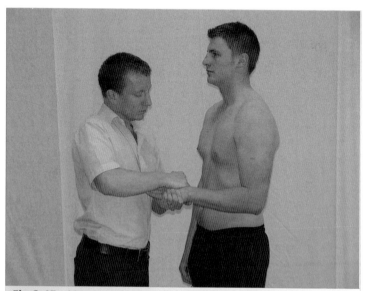

Fig 2.45 Yergason's test. The clinician positions the patient's wrist into full pronation and asks the patient to supinate the wrist.

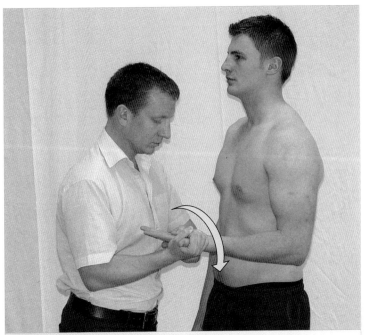

Fig 2.46 Yergason's test. The clinician resists supination and assesses for reported pain in the shoulder region.

FINDINGS

Positive result: Reported pain located over the bicipital groove area of the humerus may indicate bicipital tendon pathology. A failure to achieve movement due to pain may indicate pain inhibition. A failure to achieve movement due to weakness (+/− pain) may indicate a muscle weakness or a rupture of the long head of biceps.

Negative result: There is no pain reported and function is normal.

Table 2.18 Sensitivity and specificity values of Yergason's test

Author	Aim of study	Design	Sensitivity	Specificity
Calis et al (2000)	To investigate the diagnostic values of clinical diagnostic tests in subacromial impingement syndrome	Correlation of 120 subjects' preoperative test findings with MRI findings	37%	86.1%
Guanche & Jones (2003)	An evaluation of seven clinical tests for tears of the glenoid labrum	Correlation of 61 subjects' clinical test findings with arthroscopy findings	For SLAP lesion only 12%	For SLAP lesion only 96%
Holtby & Razmjou (2004)	Explore and describe reasons for variations in diagnostic accuracy of clinical tests in predicting biceps tendon pathology and SLAP lesions	Correlation of 152 subjects' preoperative test findings with surgical findings	43%	79%

Notes

HORIZONTAL ADDUCTION TEST

The horizontal adduction test is designed to test for acromioclavicular joint pathology; the test may also aid in the identification of impingement-type symptoms. The test is also known as the 'scarf test' or the 'cross body adduction test'. The procedure of the test involves adduction and flexion of the shoulder joint, as if wrapping a scarf over the opposite shoulder. This action applies a rotational torsion to the acromioclavicular joint and thus loads the joint structure. Furthermore, the position may act to compress the anterior aspect of the subacromial space and thus reproduce signs of impingement. An expected positive response from this test is the reproduction of the patient's pain.

PROCEDURE

Patient: The patient is positioned in standing, their shoulder adducted across their body horizontally in 90° flexion (Fig. 2.47). *Clinician:*   The clinician is standing by the patient, supporting the limb fully and therefore enabling horizontal adduction to be performed passively by the clinician, ruling out any contractile element. The clinician applies a force through the elbow to add over-pressure to the position (Fig. 2.48).

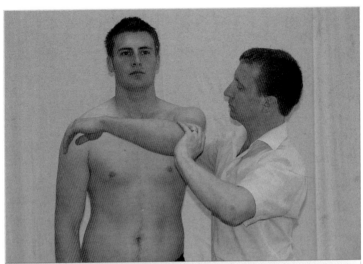

Fig 2.47   Horizontal adduction test. The clinician positions the patient into horizontal adduction.

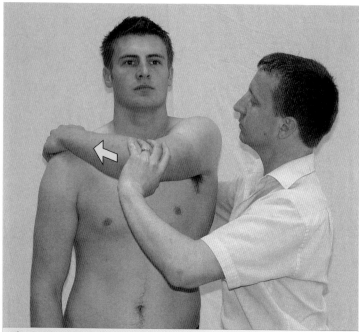

Fig 2.48 Horizontal adduction test. The clinician applies a force through the elbow and assesses for reproduction of symptoms.

FINDINGS

Positive result: Pain reported over the acromioclavicular joint as horizontal adduction occurs may suggest that the pain is arising from the acromioclavicular joint.

Negative result: There are no reported symptoms during application of the test.

Table 2.19 Sensitivity and specificity values of the horizontal adduction test

Author	Aim of study	Design	Sensitivity	Specificity
Park et al (2005)	To determine the diagnostic accuracy of clinical tests for the different degrees of subacromial impingement syndrome	Correlation of 359 subjects' preoperative test findings with arthroscopic findings	22.5%	82%

REFERENCES

Bennett W 1998 Specificity of the Speed's test: arthroscopic technique for evaluating the biceps tendon at the level of the bicipital groove. Arthroscopy 14(8): 789–796

Calis M, Akgun K, Birtane M et al 2000 Diagnostic values of clinical diagnostic tests in subacromial impingement syndrome. Annals of the Rheumatic Diseases 59(1): 44–47

Farber A, Castillo R, Clough M et al 2006 Clinical assessment of three common tests for traumatic anterior shoulder instability. Journal of Bone and Joint Surgery 88(7): 1467–1474

Gross M, Distefano M 1997 Anterior release test. Clinical Orthopaedics and Related Research 339: 105–108

Guanche C, Jones D 2003 Clinical testing for tears of the glenoid labrum. Journal of Arthroscopic and Related Surgery 19(5): 517–523

Holtby R, Razmjou H 2004 Accuracy of the Speed's and Yergason's tests in detecting biceps pathology and SLAP lesions: comparison with arthroscopic findings. Arthroscopy 20(3): 231–236

Kim S, Park J, Jeong W et al 2005 The Kim test: a novel test for posteroinferior labral lesion of the shoulder – a comparison to the jerk test. American Journal of Sports Medicine 33(8): 1188–1192

Leroux J, Thomas E, Bonnel F et al 1995 Diagnostic values of clinical tests for shoulder impingement syndrome. Revue du Rhumatism English Edition 62(6): 423–428

Lo I, Nonweiler B, Woolfrey M et al 2004 An evaluation of the apprehension, relocation and surprise tests for anterior shoulder instability. American Journal of Sports Medicine 32(2): 301–307

McFarland E, Kim T, Savino R 2002 Clinical assessment of three common tests for superior labral anterior–posterior lesions. American Journal of Sports Medicine 30(6): 810–815

O'Brien S, Pagnani M, Fealy S et al 1998 The active compression test: a new and effective test for diagnosing labral tears and acromioclavicular joint abnormality. American Journal of Sports Medicine 26(5): 610–613

Park H, Yokota A, Gill H et al 2005 Diagnostic accuracy of clinical tests for the different degrees of subacromial impingement. Journal of Bone and Joint Surgery 87(7): 1446–1455

Stetson W, Templin K 2002 The crank test, the O'Brien test and routine magnetic resonance imaging scans in the diagnosis of labral tears. American Journal of Sports Medicine 30(6): 806–809

Tzannes A, Murrell G 2002 Clinical examination of the unstable shoulder. Sports Medicine 32(7): 447–457

Walch G, Boulahia A, Calderone S et al 1998 The 'dropping' and 'Hornblower's' signs in evaluation of rotator cuff tears. Journal of Bone and Joint Surgery 80(4): 624–628

Walton J, Mahajan S, Paxinos A et al 2004 Diagnostic values of tests for acromioclavicular joint pain. Journal of Bone and Joint Surgery 86(4): 807–812

BIBLIOGRAPHY AND FURTHER READING

Gerber C, Ganz R 1984 Clinical assessment of instability of the shoulder. Journal of Bone and Joint Surgery 56(4): 551–556

Magee D 2008 Orthopedic physical assessment, 5th edn. Saunders Elsevier, St Louis, MO

Norris C 2005 Sports injuries diagnosis and management, 3rd edn. Butterworth-Heinemann, Edinburgh

Tennent D, Beach W, Meyers J 2003 A review of the special tests associated with shoulder examination part 1: The rotator cuff tests. American Journal of Sports Medicine 31(1): 154–160

Tennent D, Beach W, Meyers J 2003 A review of the special tests associated with shoulder examination part 2: Laxity, instability and superior labral anterior and posterior (SLAP) lesions. American Journal of Sports Medicine 31(2): 301–307

CHAPTER

The elbow

3

VARUS STRESS TEST

The varus stress test of the elbow is designed to test the integrity of the lateral collateral ligament of the elbow. The procedure of the test involves the clinician positioning the patient's elbow into approximately 20° flexion and applying a varus force, attempting to gap the lateral joint line of the elbow. The act of gapping the lateral joint line results in a tensioning of the lateral collateral ligament. An expected positive response from this test is an increase in the amount of gapping exhibited over the lateral joint line and/or reproduction of the patient's symptoms.

PROCEDURE

Patient: The patient is positioned in supine on a plinth. Their shoulder is in slight abduction and their elbow in approximately 20° of flexion. It is easier to perform this test standing between the patient's trunk and arm.

Clinician: The clinician is standing alongside the patient, supporting the upper arm as close to the elbow joint line as possible, without

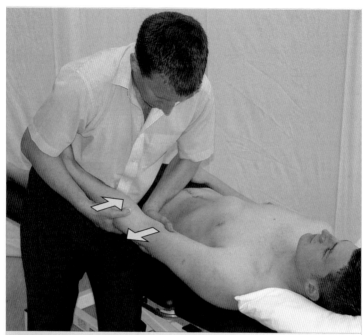

Fig 3.1 Varus stress test. The clinician positions their hands close to the joint line and applies a varus force to the elbow, gapping the lateral joint line.

impeding any possible movement. Their other hand is grasping the patient's forearm, distal to the joint line, and controlling the degree of flexion required at the elbow joint. The clinician applies the varus force and monitors the degree of laxity, and observes the patient's face for signs of discomfort (Fig. 3.1). The clinician compares the results of this side to the non-affected elbow.

FINDINGS

Positive result: Laxity and/or pain over the lateral collateral ligament of the elbow may suggest instability of the lateral collateral ligament of the elbow.

Negative result: There is no demonstration of laxity or pain on application of the test.

VALGUS STRESS TEST

The valgus stress test of the elbow is designed to test the integrity of the medial collateral ligament of the elbow. This test is also known as 'Jobe's elbow stress test'. The procedure of the test involves the clinician positioning the patient's elbow into slight flexion and applying a valgus force, attempting to gap the medial joint line of the elbow. The act of gapping the medial joint line results in a tensioning of the medial collateral ligament. An expected positive response from this test is an increase in the amount of gapping exhibited over the lateral joint line and/or reproduction of the patient's symptoms.

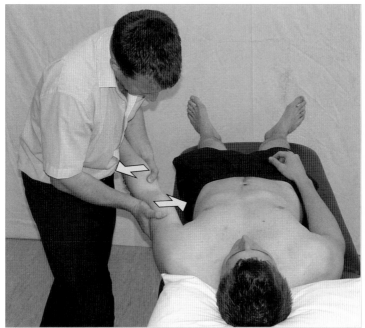

Fig 3.2 Valgus stress test. The clinician positions their hands close to the joint line and applies a valgus force to the elbow, gapping the medial joint line.

PROCEDURE
Patient: The patient is positioned in supine on a plinth. Their shoulder is in slight abduction and their elbow in approximately 20° of flexion.
Clinician: The clinician is standing alongside the patient, support-ing the upper arm above the elbow joint line, as close to the joint line as possible without impeding any possible movement. Their other hand is positioned on the medial surface of the forearm,

again as close as possible to the joint line on the medial side. The clinician then applies a gapping force to the medial joint line. The clinician applies the valgus force and monitors the degree of laxity, and observes the patient's face for signs of discomfort (Fig. 3.2). The clinician compares the results of this side to the non-affected elbow.

FINDINGS

Positive result: Laxity and/or pain over the medial collateral ligament of the elbow may suggest instability of the medial collateral ligament of the elbow.

Negative result: There is no demonstration of laxity or pain on testing.

MOVING VALGUS STRESS TEST

The moving valgus stress test is designed to test the integrity of the medial collateral ligament of the elbow. The procedure involves the clinician applying a valgus stress to the medial ligament of the elbow while performing extension and flexion of the joint. The additional movements of flexion and extension take the medial ligament through the angle of shear where the joint will be separated maximally and thus will provide a zone of maximal stress onto the ligamentous structure. This may be equated to trying to find the position where the ligament is at its greatest stretch. An expected positive response from this test is patient reported pain or symptoms in the range 70–120° flexion.

PROCEDURE

Patient: The patient is positioned in sitting on a plinth. Their shoulder is in 90° flexion/abduction, their elbow in full flexion.

Clinician: The clinician is standing in front of the patient, one hand supporting the upper arm above the elbow joint and the other hand grasping the wrist. The clinician applies a medial rotation force to the humerus while fixing the forearm at the wrist; this produces the necessary valgus stress to the medial aspect of the elbow (Fig. 3.3). The clinician then applies a flexion and extension movement to the elbow while simultaneously maintaining the valgus force (Fig. 3.4).

FINDINGS

Positive result: Pain reported as the elbow passes between 70° and 120° of flexion may suggest compromised integrity of the medial

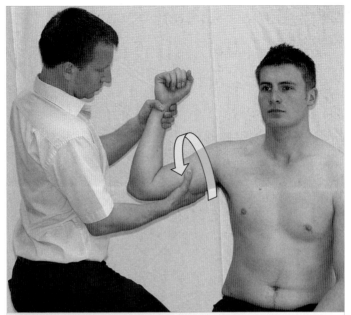

Fig 3.3 Moving valgus stress test. The clinician applies a medial rotational force to the humerus while fixing the forearm; this induces a valgus stress to the medial joint line.

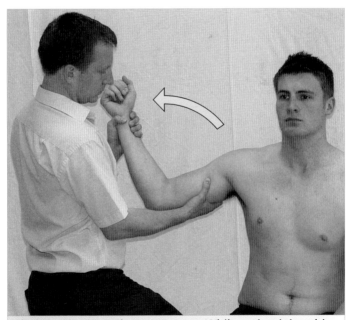

Fig 3.4 Moving valgus stress test. While maintaining this position the clinician extends and flexes the elbow and assesses for reported pain between 70° and 120° flexion.

collateral ligament. Interestingly, it is thought that the patient's pain response is worst during the flexion to extension movement rather than the extension through to flexion movement.

Negative result: No reported pain in the range 70–120° on elbow flexion or extension.

LATERAL PIVOT SHIFT TEST OF THE ELBOW

The lateral pivot shift test of the elbow is designed to test for posterolateral rotator instability of the elbow. This test is also known as the 'posterolateral rotatory instability test'. The procedure of the test involves the combination of an axial compression force, valgus stress and supination applied to the elbow. This directs the ulna to move in the posterolateral direction, the most common pattern of elbow instability. This test may be provocative for someone who has posterolateral instability of the elbow

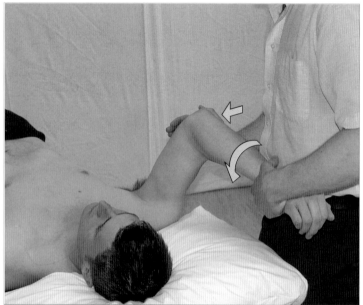

Fig 3.5 Lateral pivot shift test of the elbow. The clinician supports the arm at the elbow with one hand and applies a valgus and axial compression force with the other.

and specialist advice should be sought if there are any concerns about its application. An expected positive response from this test is a visible subluxation of the ulna from the trochlear surface of the humerus. An audible 'clunk' may also occur as the articular surfaces relocate.

PROCEDURE

Patient: The patient is positioned in supine on a plinth. Their shoulder is in approximately 160° of flexion, the elbow in 20–30° of flexion and supinated.

Clinician: The clinician is standing at the top of the plinth, one hand supporting the patient's forearm distal to the elbow joint and applying the axial force down through the line of the ulna. Their other hand is grasping the patient's wrist and applying the valgus stress to the elbow and maintaining the supinated position of the wrist (Fig. 3.5). When this position is maintained the clinician gently moves the elbow joint into further flexion (Fig. 3.6).

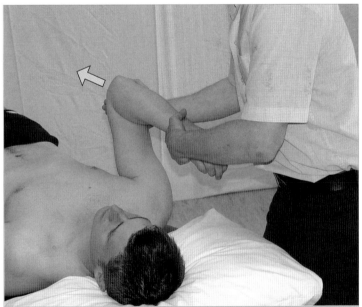

Fig 3.6 Lateral pivot shift test of the elbow. The clinician moves the elbow into further flexion and observes for a visual subluxation of the ulna on the trochlear surface.

Positive result: A visible subluxation of the humeroulnar joint, which may appear as a skin dimple occurring over the head of the radius, may suggest posterolateral instability of the elbow. The dimple arises because the skin and superficial soft tissue are sucked in behind the radial head during movement. There may also be an audible 'clunk', on relocation.
Negative result: There is no skin dimple apparent on flexion of the elbow joint and no audible 'clunk'.

RESISTED TENNIS ELBOW TEST

The resisted tennis elbow test is designed to test for tendinopathy of the common extensor origin of the elbow. The procedure involves the clinician applying resistance to the patient's attempts to extend their wrist. Wrist extension requires concentric use of the extensor origin muscles. Active contraction acts to pull through the extensor origin attached to the lateral epicondyle of the humerus. The concentric force may reproduce the patient's symptoms over the site of a lesion and thus aid in confirming the diagnosis of 'tendinopathy' of the common extensor origin. An expected positive response from this test is reproduction of the patient's pain or symptoms. The test may also identify weakness of the muscle group.

PROCEDURE
Patient: The patient is positioned in sitting or standing. Their shoulder is in 90° of flexion, their elbow in extension, their forearm pronated and their wrist in full flexion (Fig. 3.7).
Clinician: The clinician is positioned alongside the arm to be tested, resisting wrist extension with either one or two hands (Fig. 3.8).

FINDINGS
Positive result: Pain located over the lateral epicondyle of the humerus may suggest tennis elbow or tendinopathy-type symptoms. Also, possible weakness in the extensor muscles may suggest a tendinopathy or muscle weakness.
Negative result: No reproduction of pain or weakness when comparing the affected side to the non-affected elbow.

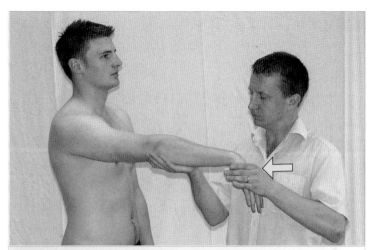

Fig 3.7 Resisted tennis elbow test. The clinician supports the arm at the elbow joint and asks the patient to extend their wrist.

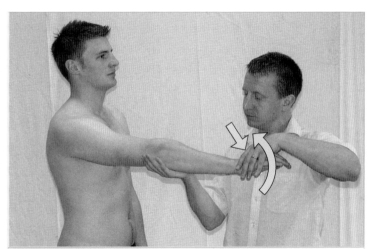

Fig 3.8 Resisted tennis elbow test. The clinician resists wrist extension and assesses for muscle weakness and reported pain.

ISOMETRIC TENNIS ELBOW TEST

The isometric tennis elbow test is designed to test for tendinopathy of the common extensor origin of the elbow. The procedure involves the clinician applying an isometric resistance to the patient's attempts to extend their wrist. An isometric contraction acts to pull through the extensor origin attached to the lateral epicondyle of the humerus. The isometric force may reproduce the patient's symptoms normally over the site of a lesion and thus aid in confirming the diagnosis of 'tendinopathy' of the common extensor origin. An expected positive response from this test is reproduction of the patient's pain or symptoms. The test may also identify weakness of the muscle group.

PROCEDURE

Patient: The patient is positioned in sitting or standing. Their shoulder is flexed to 90°, their elbow is in full extension and their wrist in neutral.

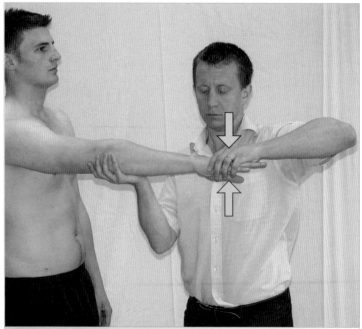

Fig 3.9   Isometric tennis elbow test. The clinician resists wrist extension isometrically.

Clinician: The clinician is positioned alongside the patient, applying an isometric resistance to the dorsum of the hand (Fig. 3.9). They can also be standing with the patient's arm positioned over their shoulder, applying an isometric resistance to the dorsum of the patient's hand.

FINDINGS

Positive result: Pain located over the lateral epicondyle of the humerus may suggest tennis elbow or tendinopathy-type symptoms. Also, possible weakness in the extensor muscles may suggest a tendinopathy or muscle weakness.

Negative result: There is no reproduction of pain or weakness when comparing the affected side to the non-affected elbow.

PASSIVE TENNIS ELBOW TEST

The passive tennis elbow test is designed to test for tendinopathy of the common extensor origin of the elbow. The procedure involves the clinician applying a passive stretch to the common extensor origin by moving the patient's wrist into full flexion. The passive stretch acts to tension the extensor origin attached to the lateral epicondyle of the humerus. The tensioning force may reproduce the patient's symptoms normally over the site of a lesion and thus aid in confirming the diagnosis of 'tendinopathy' of the common extensor origin. A potential benefit of this test, over the resisted or isometric tests, is that it removes the active component which helps to differentiate between contractile and non-contractile structure involvement. An expected positive response from this test is reproduction of the patient's pain or symptoms.

PROCEDURE

Patient: The patient is positioned in sitting or standing. Their shoulder is flexed to 90°, their elbow in full extension and their wrist passively held in full flexion and pronation (Fig. 3.10).

Clinician: The clinician is positioned alongside the patient, applying a passive stretch to the wrist flexors, to produce a stretch at the common extensor origin site (Fig. 3.11).

FINDINGS

Positive result: Pain located over the lateral epicondyle of the humerus may suggest tennis elbow or tendinopathy-type

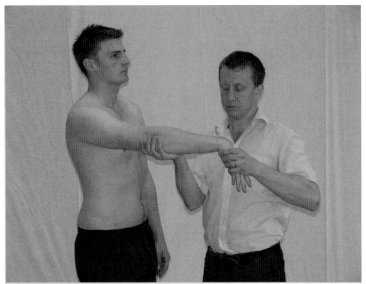

Fig 3.10 Passive tennis elbow test. The clinician supports and maintains extension at the elbow.

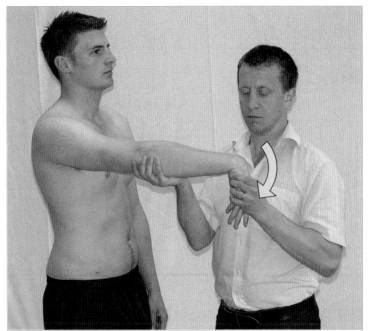

Fig 3.11 Passive tennis elbow test. The clinician applies passive wrist flexion which results in a stretch of the common extensor origin.

symptoms. Also, possible weakness in the extensor muscles may suggest a tendinopathy or muscle weakness.

Negative result: There is no reproduction of pain or weakness when comparing the affected side to the non-affected elbow.

RESISTED GOLFER'S ELBOW TEST

The resisted golfer's elbow test is designed to test for tendinopathy of the common flexor origin of the elbow. The procedure involves the clinician applying resistance to the patient's attempts to flex their wrist. Wrist flexion requires concentric use of the flexor origin muscles. Active contraction acts to pull through the flexor origin attached to the medial epicondyle of the humerus. The concentric force may reproduce the patient's symptoms normally over the site of a lesion and thus aid in confirming the diagnosis of 'tendinopathy' of the common flexor origin. An expected positive response from this test is reproduction of the

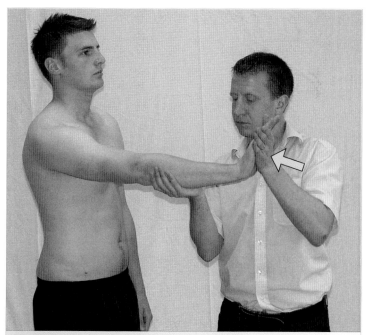

Fig 3.12   Resisted golfer's elbow test. The clinician supports the arm at the elbow joint and asks the patient to flex their wrist.

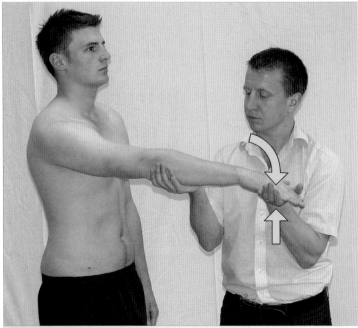

Fig 3.13 Resisted golfer's elbow test. The clinician resists wrist flexion and assesses for muscle weakness and reported pain.

patient's pain or symptoms. The test may also identify weakness of the muscle group.

PROCEDURE

Patient: The patient is positioned in sitting or standing. Their shoulder is in 90° of flexion, with the elbow in extension, the forearm pronated and the wrist in full extension (Fig. 3.12).

Clinician: The clinician is positioned alongside the arm to be tested, if the patient is sitting, resisting wrist flexion with either one or two hands (Fig. 3.13).

FINDINGS

Positive result: Pain located over the medial epicondyle of the humerus may suggest golfer's elbow or tendinopathy-type symptoms. Also, possible weakness in the flexor muscles may suggest a tendinopathy or muscle weakness.

Negative result: There is no reproduction of pain or weakness when comparing the affected side to the non-affected elbow.

ISOMETRIC GOLFER'S ELBOW TEST

The isometric golfer's elbow test is designed to test for tendinopathy of the common flexor origin of the elbow. The procedure involves the clinician applying an isometric resistance to the patient's attempts to flex their wrist. An isometric contraction acts to pull through the flexor origin attached to the medial epicondyle of the humerus. The isometric force may reproduce the patient's symptoms normally over the site of a lesion and thus aid in confirming the diagnosis of 'tendinopathy' of the common flexor origin. An expected positive response from this test is reproduction of patient's pain or symptoms. The test may also identify weakness of the muscle group.

PROCEDURE

Patient: The patient is positioned in sitting or standing. Their shoulder is flexed to 90°, with the elbow in full extension and the wrist in neutral.

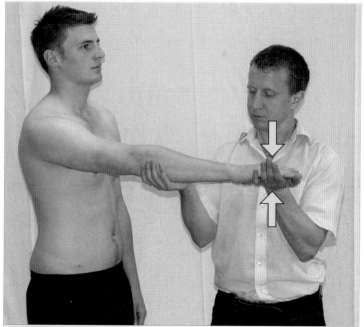

Fig 3.14   Isometric golfer's elbow test. The clinician resists wrist flexion isometrically.

Clinician: The clinician is positioned alongside the patient, applying an isometric resistance to the palmar surface of the hand (Fig. 3.14).

FINDINGS

Positive result: Pain located over the medial epicondyle of the humerus may suggest golfer's elbow or tendinopathy-type symptoms. Also, possible weakness in the flexor muscles may suggest a tendinopathy or muscle weakness.

Negative result: There is no reproduction of pain or weakness when comparing the affected side to the non-affected elbow.

PASSIVE GOLFER'S ELBOW TEST

The passive golfer's elbow test is designed to test for tendinopathy of the common flexor origin of the elbow. The procedure involves the clinician applying a passive stretch to the common flexor origin by moving the patient's wrist into full extension. The passive stretch acts to tension the flexor origin attached to the medial epicondyle of the humerus. The tensioning force may reproduce the patient's symptoms normally over the site of a lesion and thus aid in confirming the diagnosis of 'tendinopathy' of the common flexor origin. A potential benefit of this test, over the resisted or isometric tests, is that it removes the active component, which helps to differentiate between contractile and non-contractile structure involvement. An expected positive response from this test is reproduction of patient's pain or symptoms.

PROCEDURE

Patient: The patient is positioned in sitting or standing. Their shoulder is flexed to 90°, their elbow is in full extension, and their wrist is held in full passive extension and supination (Fig. 3.15).

Clinician: The clinician is positioned alongside the patient, applying a passive stretch to the wrist flexors, to produce a stretch at the common flexor origin site (Fig. 3.16).

FINDINGS

Positive result: Pain located over the medial epicondyle of the humerus may suggest golfer's elbow or tendinopathy-type symptoms. Also, possible weakness in the flexor muscles may suggest a tendinopathy or muscle weakness.

Negative result: There is no reproduction of pain or weakness when comparing the affected side to the non-affected elbow.

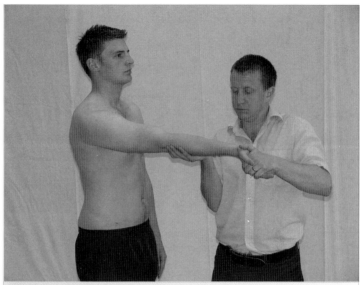

Fig 3.15 Passive golfer's elbow test. The clinician supports and maintains extension at the elbow.

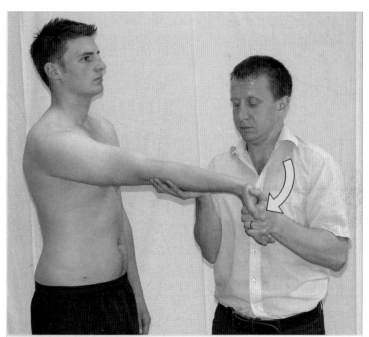

Fig 3.16 Passive golfer's elbow test. The clinician applies passive wrist extension which results in a stretch of the common flexor origin.

ELBOW FLEXION TEST

The elbow flexion test is designed to test the integrity of the ulnar nerve at the cubital tunnel. The procedure of the test involves applying a compression force onto the ulnar nerve at the elbow by the clinician positioning the patient into sustained elbow flexion for 3 minutes. Compression of a nerve may lead to the reproduction of nerve-oriented symptoms, such as pain, numbness, tingling or pins and needles. As the elbow is flexed it is thought the ulnar nerve is compressed somewhere between the medial epicondyle of the humerus and the olecranon. Additional wrist flexion is thought to also add a possible traction force and thus lead to a possible ischaemic episode to the ulnar nerve at the elbow. An expected positive response from this test is the reproduction of the patient's symptoms.

PROCEDURE

Patient: The patient is positioned in sitting. Both elbows are fully flexed, but not forcibly flexed or held. The forearms are fully supinated and the wrists relaxed or positioned in full flexion (Fig. 3.17).

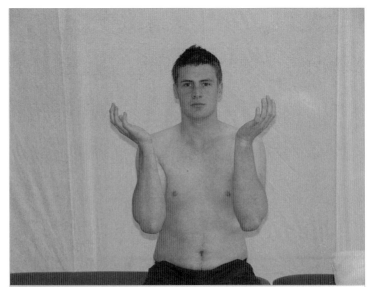

Fig 3.17   Elbow flexion test. The patient maintains elbow flexion for 3 minutes while the clinician monitors for reproduction of symptoms at designated time intervals.

Clinician: The clinician monitors the patient's symptoms by asking them, at designated time intervals (normally 15, 30, 60, 125 and 180 seconds) after positioning, if there is any change in or reproduction of their symptoms.

FINDINGS

Positive result: The onset of pain, numbness and/or tingling within the maximum time of 3 minutes may suggest the ulnar nerve has been sensitized and thus the traction has led to an ischaemic episode in the nerve that has produced their symptoms.
Negative result: There is no reproduction of pain, numbness or tingling.

PRONATOR TERES TEST

The pronator teres test is designed to test for potential entrapment of the median nerve at the elbow. The procedure of the test involves the clinician resisting isometric pronation of the elbow by the patient. This action leads to an isometric contraction of pronator teres. The median nerve passes from the upper arm to the forearm between the two heads of pronator teres and thus the contraction causes compression or entrapment of the nerve at this point. An expected positive response from this test is the reproduction of pronator teres syndrome symptoms, which are typically numbness or tingling along the path of the median nerve.

PROCEDURE

Patient: The patient is standing or sitting. Their shoulder is in slight flexion, with their elbow in 90° of flexion, forearm supinated and wrist in neutral (Fig. 3.18).
Clinician: The clinician is positioned in front of the patient, supporting the patient's elbow. One hand is grasping the patient's outstretched hand as if to shake hands, but maintaining the patient's supinated position. The clinician asks the patient to try and turn their hand over, so the palm is facing downwards. The clinician resists this movement isometrically, so there is no resultant movement (Fig. 3.19). The clinician can also extend the patient's elbow during the application of the isometric resistance. Note that the patient must not try and resist the additional extension to the elbow, as this could potentially incorporate other adjacent muscle activity.

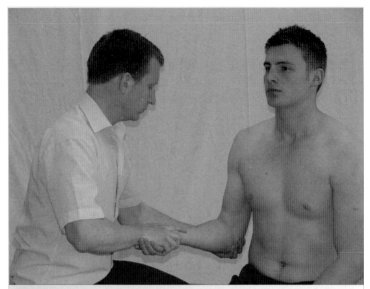

Fig 3.18 Pronator teres test. The clinician supports the elbow and grasps the patient's hand in full supination.

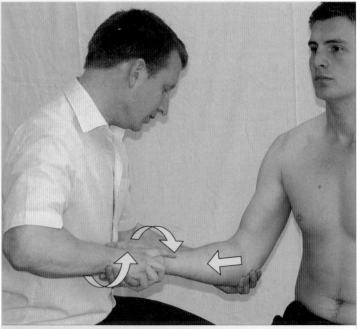

Fig 3.19 Pronator teres test. The clinician resists pronation while slowly extending the patient's elbow.

FINDINGS

Positive result: Reproduction of the patient's pain or initiation of nerve-oriented symptoms; for example, numbness or tingling along a median nerve distribution may indicate that the isometric activity of resisting pronator teres has led to a type of compression or impingement of the median nerve.

Negative result: There is no reproduction of symptoms or further production of nerve-oriented symptoms.

PINCH GRIP TEST

The pinch grip test is designed to test for potential entrapment of the anterior interosseous branch of the median nerve. The procedure of the test involves the patient forming a pinch grip with their index finger and thumb. The anterior interosseous branch of the median nerve supplies flexor pollicis longus, flexor digitorum profundus (lateral part) and pronator quadratus. The formation of a pinch grip therefore uses flexor pollicis longus and flexor digitorum profundus. The anterior interosseous branch splits off the main trunk of the median nerve at the exit point of the nerve, passing through pronator teres. Even though it is located close to the median nerve, there is a slight difference in a patient's presentation if it is compressed when compared to the median nerve. The anterior interosseous branch has only a motor supply with no sensory innervation, whereas the median nerve has both motor and sensory roles. Therefore the pinch grip test may help in differentiating between a compression of the median nerve and the anterior interosseous branch. An expected positive result of this test is the failure to maintain a tip-to-tip pinch grip of the thumb and index finger. The test may also indicate signs of muscle weakness.

PROCEDURE

Patient: The patient is positioned in sitting or standing.

Clinician: The clinician instructs the patient to form a pinch grip between their thumb and their index finger (Fig. 3.20).

FINDINGS

Positive result: The patient is unable to form a tip-to-tip link between the thumb and index finger, with an inability to prevent the distal interphalangeal joint from extending, leading to a pad-to-pad contact of the thumb and finger, rather than finger tip to finger tip (Fig. 3.21).

Negative result: A firm grip between the thumb and index finger.

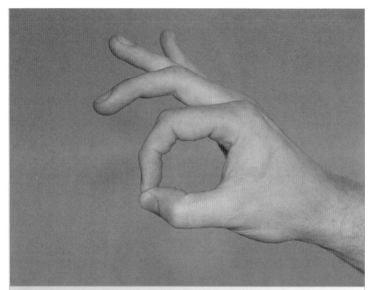

Fig 3.20 Pinch grip test. The patient attempts to form a pinch grip between their thumb and index finger.

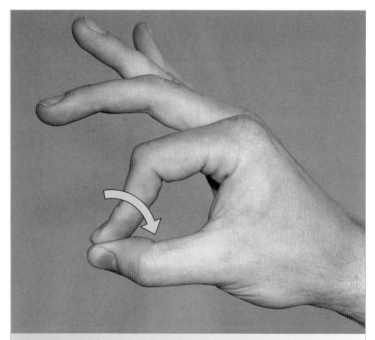

Fig 3.21 Pinch grip test. Failure to maintain a tip-to-tip contact indicates a positive result.

NB 1 Clinically, you may see the 'strength' of the contact between the thumb and finger being tested by the clinician, linking their finger and thumb around the patient's and attempting to break the loop.

NB 2 Secondly, this test is often confused with the Froment's sign test (see Ch. 4). Even though the action of the test is similar, the context of what is being tested is different. The pinch grip test is used to investigate the anterior interosseous nerve integrity (median nerve) around the elbow, while Froment's sign test is concerned with possible ulnar nerve integrity around the wrist joint, since the flexor digitorum profundus is supplied by both the median and ulnar nerves.

BIBLIOGRAPHY AND FURTHER READING

Buehler M, Thayer D 1988 The elbow flexion test: a clinical test for the cubital tunnel syndrome. Clinical Orthopaedics and Related Research 233: 213–216

Magee D 2008 Orthopedic physical assessment, 5th edn. Saunders Elsevier, St Louis, MO

Norris C 2005 Sports injuries diagnosis and management, 3rd edn. Butterworth-Heinemann, Edinburgh

O'Driscoll S 2000 Classification and evaluation of recurrent instability of the elbow. Clinical Orthopaedics and Related Research 370: 34–43

O'Driscoll S, Morrey B 1991 Posterolateral rotator instability of the elbow. Journal of Bone and Joint Surgery 73(3): 440–446

O'Driscoll S, Lawton R, Smith A 2005 The 'moving valgus stress test' for medial collateral ligament tears of the elbow. American Journal of Sports Medicine 33(2): 231–239

Notes

The wrist and hand

ULNOCARPAL STRESS TEST

The ulnocarpal stress test is designed to test the stability of the wrist joint, in particular the triangular fibrocartilage complex of the wrist. This test is also known as 'McMurray's test of the wrist'. The procedure of the test involves the clinician applying a compressive force through the wrist joint while moving the wrist from an ulna deviated, supinated position to a pronated position. Ulnar deviation acts to compress the space between the distal end of the ulna and the triquetral, situated in the proximal row of carpal bones. Combined with a rotational movement, the action may impinge soft tissue structures situated within the joint complex. An expected positive response from this test is an audible 'click' within the joint as the articular structures compress and grind the triangular fibrocartilage complex. The test may also act to reproduce the patient's symptoms.

PROCEDURE
Patient: The patient is positioned in sitting. Their elbow is fully flexed, with the wrist in full active ulnar deviation and the forearm in supination (Fig. 4.1).

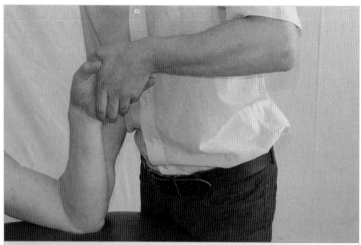

Fig 4.1   Ulnocarpal stress test. The clinician supports the elbow and applies ulnar deviation, compressing the triangular fibrocartilage complex in a supinated position.

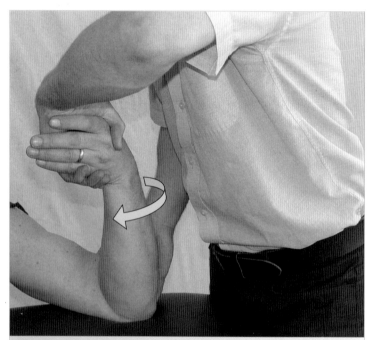

Fig 4.2   Ulnocarpal stress test. While maintaining ulnar deviation the clinician pronates the wrist and assesses for an audible 'click' and reported pain.

Clinician: The clinician is standing alongside the patient, supporting the patient's elbow. The clinician grasps the palm of the patient's hand and can then maintain the ulnar deviation and produce the movement of supination to pronation (Fig. 4.2).

FINDINGS

Positive result: An audible 'click' during the application of the test, together with pain on the medial aspect of the wrist within the ulnocarpal region, may suggest potential instability of the ulnocarpal complex. Interestingly, a 'click' without the presence of pain should not necessarily be considered a positive result.

Negative result: There is no reproduction of the symptoms. There may be an audible 'click', but with no pain.

LUNOTRIQUETRAL BALLOTTEMENT TEST

The lunotriquetral ballottement test is designed to test for the integrity of the lunotriquetral ligament complex. This test is also known as 'Reagan's test'. The procedure of the test involves applying a shearing force between the lunate and the triquetral. The clinician applies an anterior to posterior force through the lunate and a posterior to anterior force through the triquetral. The resultant shearing force acts to tension the lunotriquetral ligament and thus tests its integrity. An expected positive response from this test is an audible 'click' as the carpal bones move. The test may also act to reproduce the patient's symptoms.

PROCEDURE

Patient: The patient is positioned in sitting, their hand supported by the clinician.

Clinician: The clinician is standing alongside the patient, positioned so they are able to apply pressure along the desired line of force. The finger and thumb of one hand isolate the lunate and the finger and thumb of the other hand isolate the triquetral. The clinician applies an anterior to posterior force to the lunate and a posterior to anterior force through the triquetral (Fig. 4.3).

FINDINGS

Positive result: An audible 'click' accompanied by pain may suggest a lunotriquetral ligament tear. Pain and crepitus may also be felt within the joint, which may also indicate a possible tear

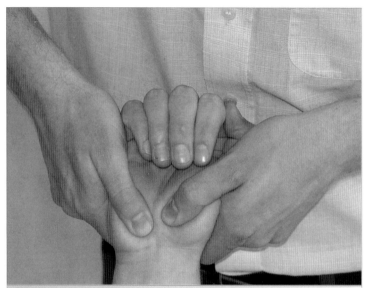

Fig 4.3 Lunotriquetral ballottement test. The clinician applies an anterior to posterior force through the lunate and a posterior to anterior force through the triquetral.

of the lunotriquetral ligament. It is possible that degeneration of the articular surfaces may result in crepitus. Further information may be perceived by comparing the range of movement available between the two bones during the applied accessory movement, when compared to the non-affected hand.

Negative result: There is no audible 'click' or reproduction of symptoms.

SCAPHOID SHIFT TEST

The scaphoid shift test is designed to test for instability of the scaphoid. This test is also known as the 'Watson test'. The procedure involves the clinician applying an anterior to posterior force to the scaphoid while performing passive radial deviation of the wrist. This action acts to compress or tension soft tissue structures around the scaphoid that would normally maintain its stability. An expected positive response from this test is an audible 'click' with or without pain. The test may also demonstrate a subluxation of the scaphoid.

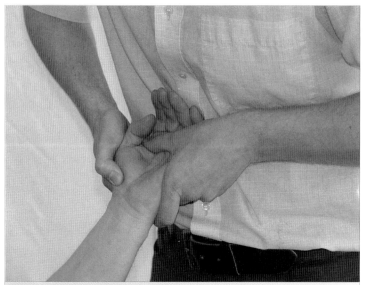

Fig 4.4 Scaphoid shift test. The clinician applies an anterior to posterior force through the scaphoid and radially deviates the wrist.

PROCEDURE

Patient: The patient is positioned in sitting, with their arm resting comfortably on a table.

Clinician: The clinician is standing by the patient. The clinician identifies the scaphoid within the anatomical snuff box and applies an anterior force, through the palmar surface, to the tubercle of the scaphoid. The clinician then applies radial deviation to the patient's wrist (Fig. 4.4).

FINDINGS

Positive result: An audible 'click' or 'pop' accompanied by pain may indicate scaphoid instability. The literature also suggests that a possible subluxation of the scaphoid is also a positive finding.

Negative result: There is no audible 'click' and/or reproduction of symptoms.

GRIND TEST

The grind test is designed to test for instability and/or degeneration of the trapeziometacarpal joint. The procedure of the test involves the clinician applying a compressive force of the base of the first metacarpal against the trapezium. The compression force acts to load the articular surfaces and thus potentially reproduce the patient's pain if arising from an articular component. An expected positive response from this test is the reproduction of the patient's pain and/or signs of degeneration, such as crepitus or clicking.

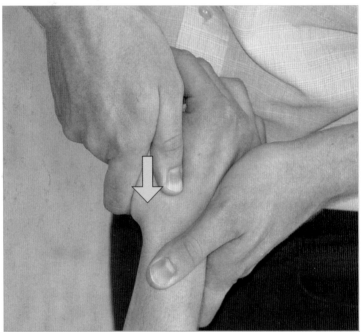

Fig 4.5   Grind test. The clinician stabilizes the wrist joint and applies a compression force down through the trapeziometacarpal joint.

PROCEDURE

Patient: The patient is positioned in sitting. Their arm is resting comfortably on a table.

Clinician: The clinician is standing by the patient, grasping the proximal phalanx and metacarpal and supporting the wrist joint (Fig. 4.5). The clinician directs a compression force down through the line of the metacarpal and adds a medial and lateral rotational component (Fig. 4.6).

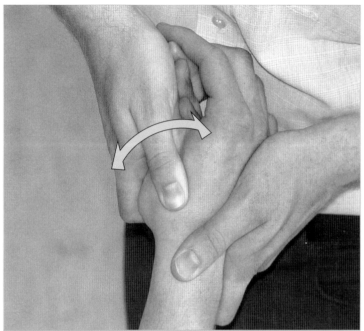

Fig 4.6 Grind test. In this position the clinician adds medial and lateral rotation to the joint and assesses for reproduction of symptoms.

FINDINGS
Positive result: Pain and/or clicking and/or crepitus during application of the test may suggest there is an element of degeneration and/or instability of the trapeziometacarpal joint.
Negative result: There is no pain, clicking or crepitus.

PHALEN'S TEST

'Phalen's test' is designed to test for carpal tunnel syndrome. This test is also known as the 'wrist flexion test'. The procedure involves positioning the patient's wrist into full passive flexion, with the aim of providing a compressive force for 60 seconds to the median nerve as it passes through the carpal bones at the wrist. Compression of the median nerve is thought to highlight an irritated or sensitized nerve and thus result in a reproduction of carpal tunnel symptoms. An expected positive response from this test is the reproduction of carpal tunnel-type symptoms, which may include tingling or pins and needles.

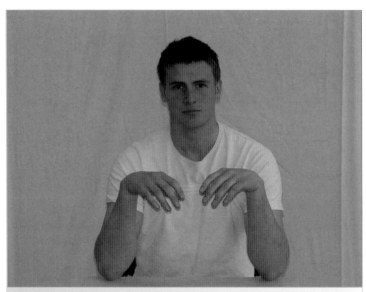

Fig 4.7 Phalen's test. The patient is positioned into passive unforced wrist flexion for 60 seconds.

PROCEDURE

Patient: The patient is positioned in sitting. Both elbows are resting on a table. The wrists are allowed to drop into full unforced flexion (Fig. 4.7).

Clinician: The clinician stands by the patient, ensuring they are positioned correctly, and times the wrist position for the duration of 60 seconds.

FINDINGS

Positive result: Reported onset of tingling, burning, pins and needles or numbness over the lateral aspect of the hand (median nerve supply) within 60 seconds may indicate a compressive element to the median nerve and suggest a diagnosis of carpal tunnel syndrome.

Negative result: There is no reported tingling, burning, pins and needles or numbness over the lateral aspect of the hand (median nerve supply) within 60 seconds.

Table 4.1 Sensitivity and specificity values of Phalen's test

Author	Aim of study	Design	Sensitivity	Specificity
Amirfeyz et al (2005)	To investigate the sensitivity and specificity of the hand elevation test, Phalen's test and Tinel's test	Correlation of 46 subjects' Phalen's test findings with post-surgical outcome findings	83%	98%
Brüske et al (2002)	To evaluate the sensitivity and specificity of the Phalen's test and Hoffmann–Tinel sign in the diagnosis of carpal tunnel syndrome	Correlation of 212 subjects' Phalen's test findings with nerve conduction test findings	85%	89%
Kuhlman & Hennessey (1997)	To determine the sensitivity and specificity of six clinical tests used to determine the presence or absence of carpal tunnel syndrome	Correlation of 180 subjects' Phalen's test findings with electrodiagnostic findings	51%	76%
LaJoie et al (2005)	To determine the accuracy rates of Tinel signs, Phalen's test and nerve conduction tests	Latent class analysis of 81 subjects' Phalen's test findings and nerve conduction test findings	92%	88%
MacDermid & Wessel (2004)	To examine the properties of the clinical tests used in the diagnosis of carpal tunnel syndrome	Systematic review of 15 studies that met the selection criteria	68% (estimate)	73% (estimate)

(table continues)

Table 4.1 (continued)

Author	Aim of study	Design	Sensitivity	Specificity
Massy-Westropp et al (2000)	To review the literature relating to the common clinical procedures used to diagnose carpal tunnel syndrome	Systematic review of seven studies that met the selection criteria.	Range 43–86%	Range 48–67%
Tetro et al (1998)	To investigate the sensitivity and specificity of the median nerve compression test, Phalen's test and Tinel's test	Correlation of 64 subjects' Phalen's test findings with nerve conduction test findings	61%	83%

PHALEN'S TEST II

'Phalen's test II' is designed to test for carpal tunnel syndrome. This test is also known as the 'forced wrist flexion test'. The procedure involves positioning the patient's wrist into forced full passive flexion by placing the dorsal surfaces of the hands together, with the aim of providing a compressive force for 60 seconds to the median nerve as it passes through the carpal bones at the wrist. Compression of the median nerve is thought to highlight an irritated or sensitized nerve and thus result in a reproduction of carpal tunnel symptoms. An expected positive response from this test is reproduction of carpal tunnel-type symptoms, which may include tingling or pins and needles.

PROCEDURE

Patient: The patient is positioned in sitting. The dorsal surfaces of their hands are placed against each other, thus forcing the wrists into flexion (Fig. 4.8).

Clinician: The clinician stands alongside the patient, ensuring they are positioned correctly, and times the wrist position for the duration of 60 seconds.

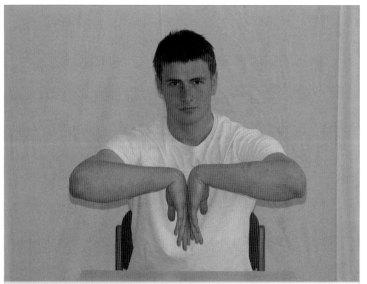

Fig 4.8 Phalen's test II. The patient is positioned into full forced wrist flexion for 60 seconds.

FINDINGS

Positive result: Reported onset of tingling, burning, pins and needles or numbness over the lateral aspect of the hand (median nerve supply) within 60 seconds. This may indicate a compressive element to the median nerve and may suggest a diagnosis of carpal tunnel syndrome.

Negative result: There is no tingling, burning, pins and needles or numbness over the lateral aspect of the hand (median nerve supply) within 60 seconds.

REVERSE PHALEN'S TEST

The reversed Phalen's test is designed to test for carpal tunnel syndrome. This test is also known as the 'wrist extension test'. The procedure involves positioning the patient's wrist into full passive extension, with the aim of providing a traction force for 120 seconds to the median nerve as it passes through the carpal bones at the wrist. Traction of the median nerve is thought to highlight an irritated or sensitized nerve and thus result in a reproduction of carpal tunnel symptoms. An expected positive

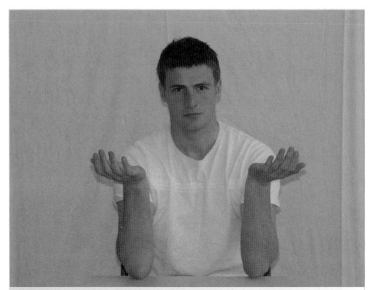

Fig 4.9 Reverse Phalen's test. The patient is positioned into passive unforced wrist extension for 120 seconds.

response from this test is reproduction of carpal tunnel-type symptoms, which may include tingling or pins and needles.

PROCEDURE

Patient: The patient is positioned in sitting. Both elbows are resting on a table. The wrists are positioned in full but not forced extension (Fig. 4.9).

Clinician: The clinician stands alongside the patient, ensuring they are positioned correctly, and times the wrist position for the duration of 120 seconds.

FINDINGS

Positive result: Reported onset of tingling, burning, pins and needles or numbness over the lateral aspect of the hand (median nerve supply) within 120 seconds may indicate a compressive element to the median nerve and may suggest a diagnosis of carpal tunnel syndrome.

Negative result: There is no tingling, burning, pins and needles or numbness over the lateral aspect of the hand (median nerve supply) within 120 seconds.

Table 4.2 Sensitivity and specificity values of the reverse Phalen's test

Author	Aim of study	Design	Sensitivity	Specificity
Massy-Westropp et al (2000)	To review the literature relating to the common clinical procedures used to diagnose carpal tunnel syndrome	Systematic review of one study that met the selection criteria	55%	100%

REVERSE PHALEN'S TEST II

The reverse Phalen's test II is designed to test for carpal tunnel syndrome. This test is also known as the 'forced wrist extension test'. The procedure involves positioning the patient's wrist into forced full passive extension by placing the palmar surfaces of the hands together, with the aim of providing a traction force for 120 seconds to the median nerve as it passes through the carpal bones at the wrist. Traction of the median nerve is thought to highlight an irritated or sensitized nerve and thus result in a reproduction of carpal tunnel symptoms. An expected positive response from this test is reproduction of carpal tunnel-type symptoms, which may include tingling or pins and needles.

PROCEDURE
Patient: The patient is positioned in sitting, with both elbows resting on a table in front of them. Their wrists are positioned in full extension, with the palmar surfaces of the hands together; thus, as they are pushed together, both wrists are forced into full 'forced' extension (Fig. 4.10).
Clinician: The clinician stands by the patient, ensuring they are positioned correctly, and times the wrist position for the duration of 120 seconds.

FINDINGS
Positive result: Reported onset of tingling, burning, pins and needles or numbness over the lateral aspect of the hand (median nerve supply) within 120 seconds may indicate a compressive element to the median nerve and may suggest a diagnosis of carpal tunnel syndrome.

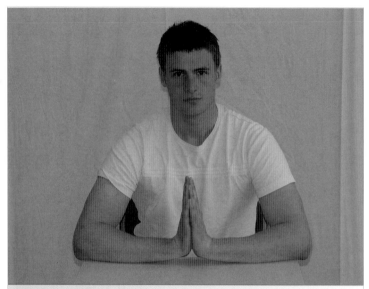

Fig 4.10 Reverse Phalen's test II. The patient is positioned into full forced wrist extension for 120 seconds.

Negative result: There is no tingling, burning, pins and needles or numbness over the lateral aspect of the hand (median nerve supply) within 120 seconds.

TINEL'S TEST

Tinel's test is designed to test for carpal tunnel syndrome. This test is also known as the 'Hoffmann–Tinel sign'. The procedure of the test involves the clinician tapping their finger directly over the path of the patient's median nerve as it passes through the carpal bones on the anterior surface of the wrist. The action of tapping the wrist is thought to produce a vibration force through the superficial tissues to the sensitized nerve; this may result in the reproduction of the patient's symptoms. There is controversy within clinical practice and the available literature as to whether a specific number of taps should be applied (10), or whether the clinician should tap for a set duration of time (30 seconds). An expected positive response from this test is the reproduction of the carpal tunnel-type symptoms, which may include tingling or pins and needles.

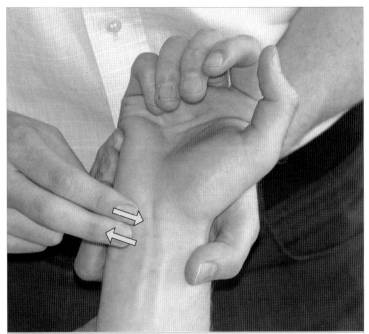

Fig 4.11 Tinel's test. The clinician taps over the path of the median nerve as it passes through the carpal bones and assesses for symptom reproduction.

PROCEDURE

Patient: The patient is positioned in sitting with the elbow supinated and the wrist positioned on a table and supported by the clinician.

Clinician: The clinician is positioned in front of the patient, applying a tapping movement, with the pads of either one or two fingers, over the path of the median nerve (Fig. 4.11).

FINDINGS

Positive result: Reported tingling over the median nerve distribution of the hand may indicate a compressive element of the median nerve at the carpal bones and thus may suggest a diagnosis of carpal tunnel syndrome. Some literature suggests that the tingling should be non-painful, others fail to specify. Alternatively, reproduction of symptoms is also identified as a positive result.

Negative result: There is no tingling or reproduction of the patient's symptoms.

Table 4.3 Sensitivity and specificity values of Tinel's test

Author	Aim of study	Design	Sensitivity	Specificity
Amirfeyz et al (2005)	To investigate the sensitivity and specificity of the hand elevation test, Phalen's test and Tinel's test	Correlation of 46 subjects' Tinel's test findings with post-surgical outcome findings	48%	94%
Brüske et al (2002)	To evaluate the sensitivity and specificity of the Phalen's test and Hoffmann–Tinel sign in the diagnosis of carpal tunnel syndrome	Correlation of 212 subjects' Tinel's test findings with nerve conduction test findings	67%	68%
Kuhlman & Hennessey (1997)	To determine the sensitivity and specificity of six clinical tests used to determine the presence or absence of carpal tunnel syndrome	Correlation of 180 subjects' Tinel's test findings with electrodiagnostic findings	23%	87%
LaJoie et al (2005)	To determine the accuracy rates of Tinel signs, Phalen's test and nerve conduction tests	Latent class analysis of 81 subjects' Tinel's test findings and nerve conduction test findings	97%	91%
MacDermid & Wessel (2004)	To examine the properties of the clinical tests used in the diagnosis of carpal tunnel syndrome	Systematic review of 15 studies that met the selection criteria	50% (estimate)	77% (estimate)

(table continues)

Table 4.3 (continued)

Author	Aim of study	Design	Sensitivity	Specificity
Massy-Westropp et al (2000)	To review the literature relating to the common clinical procedures used to diagnose carpal tunnel syndrome	Systematic review of seven studies that met the selection criteria	Range 45–75%	Range 40–67%
Tetro et al (1998)	To investigate the sensitivity and specificity of the median nerve compression test, Phalen's test and Tinel's test	Correlation of 64 subjects' Tinel's test findings with nerve conduction test findings	74%	91%

CARPAL COMPRESSION TEST

The carpal compression test is designed to test for carpal tunnel syndrome. This test is also known as the 'median nerve compression test' and the 'Durkan test'. The procedure involves the clinician compressing the median nerve as it passes through the carpal bones by grasping the wrist. Compression of an already compressed or sensitized nerve may lead to further sensitization and thus result in symptom provocation. An expected positive response from this test is the reproduction of the carpal tunnel-type symptoms, which may include tingling or pins and needles.

PROCEDURE

Patient: The patient is positioned in sitting. Their elbow is supinated, with the wrist in neutral and the forearm supported by the clinician.

Clinician: The clinician is standing by the patient, applying moderate pressure over the median nerve, above or just distal to the distal wrist crease. The pressure is maintained for 5 seconds (Fig. 4.12).

FINDINGS

Positive result: Pain and paraesthesia in the hand in the median nerve distribution may suggest carpal tunnel syndrome. Clinically, if the patient's symptoms are reproduced, this may also be considered a positive finding.

Negative result: There is no pain, paraesthesia or reproduction of the patient's symptoms.

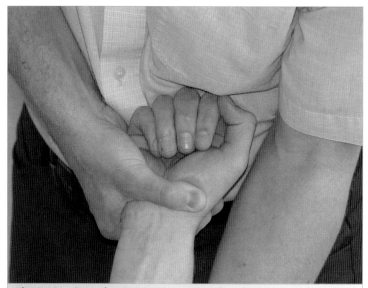

Fig 4.12 Carpal compression test. The clinician applies compression to the patient's wrist for 5 seconds and monitors for symptom reproduction.

Table 4.4 Sensitivity and specificity values of the carpal compression test

Author	Aim of study	Design	Sensitivity	Specificity
Kuhlman & Hennessey (1997)	To determine the sensitivity and specificity of six clinical tests used to determine the presence of carpal tunnel syndrome	Correlation of 180 subjects' median compression test findings with electrodiagnostic findings	28%	74%

(table continues)

Table 4.4 (continued)

Author	Aim of study	Design	Sensitivity	Specificity
MacDermid & Wessel (2004)	To examine the properties of the clinical tests used in the diagnosis of carpal tunnel syndrome	Systematic review of 15 studies that met the selection criteria	64% (estimated)	83% (estimated)
Massy-Westropp et al (2000)	To review the literature relating to the common clinical procedures used to diagnose carpal tunnel syndrome	Systematic review of three studies that met the selection criteria	Range 49–89%	Range 54–96%
Tetro et al (1998)	To investigate the sensitivity and specificity of the median nerve compression test, Phalen's test and Tinel's test	Correlation of 64 subjects' median compression test findings with nerve conduction test findings	75%	93%

WRIST FLEXION AND COMPRESSION TEST

The wrist flexion and compression test is designed to test for carpal tunnel syndrome. The procedure of the test involves the clinician positioning the patient's wrist in 60° of flexion and applying a compressive force over the path of the median nerve at the wrist. This test combines the effects of Phalen's test and the carpal compression test. This combination may increase the effect of compression on to the median nerve, thus resulting in a stronger mechanical effect. An expected positive response from this test is the reproduction of the carpal tunnel-type symptoms, which may include tingling or pins and needles.

PROCEDURE
Patient: The patient is positioned in sitting. Their elbow is positioned in full extension and full supination.

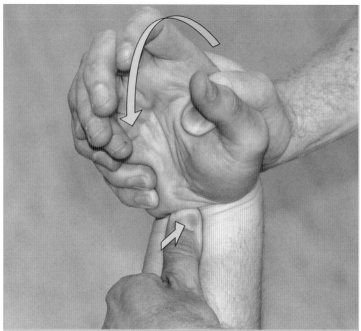

Fig 4.13 Wrist flexion and compression test. The clinician applies pressure over the path of the median nerve while maintaining wrist flexion for 30 seconds.

Clinician: The clinician is standing by the patient, placing the wrist to be tested in 60° of flexion, as well as applying their thumb on to the path of the median nerve as it passes through the wrist joint. After applying the wrist flexion and compression, the clinician records the time taken until the symptoms occur (Fig. 4.13).

FINDINGS

Positive result: Reproduction of the patient's symptoms within 30 seconds may suggest carpal tunnel syndrome.

Negative result: There is no reproduction of symptoms associated with carpal tunnel after 30 seconds of the test duration.

Table 4.5 Sensitivity and specificity values of the wrist flexion and compression test

Author	Aim of study	Design	Sensitivity	Specificity
Massy-Westropp et al (2000)	To review the literature relating to the common clinical procedures used to diagnose carpal tunnel syndrome	Systematic review of one study that met the selection criteria	82%	99%
Tetro et al (1998)	To investigate the sensitivity and specificity of the median nerve compression test, Phalen's test and Tinel's test	Correlation of 64 subjects' wrist flexion and compression test findings with nerve conduction test findings	86%	95%

HAND ELEVATION TEST

The hand elevation test is designed to test for carpal tunnel syndrome. The procedure of the test involves the patient elevating their arm as high as possible above their head. Elevation of the limb may act to traction or compress the brachial plexus neural network, and thus create a transmitted force that may highlight an irritated or sensitized median nerve, and thus result in a reproduction of carpal tunnel symptoms. An expected positive response from this test is the reproduction of the carpal tunnel-type symptoms, which may include tingling or pins and needles.

PROCEDURE

Patient: The patient is positioned in sitting. Their arm is elevated as high above their head as possible, for 1 minute's duration (Fig. 4.14).

Clinician: The clinician stands by the patient, instructing them in the correct procedure and timing the clinical test.

FINDINGS

Positive result: Reproduction of the patient's symptoms within 1 minute may suggest carpal tunnel syndrome.

Negative result: There is no reproduction of the symptoms after 1 minute.

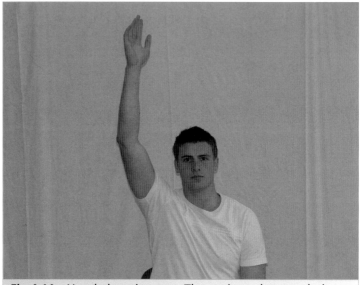

Fig 4.14 Hand elevation test. The patient elevates their arm above their head for 1 minute while the clinician assesses for symptom reproduction.

Table 4.6 Sensitivity and specificity values of the hand elevation test

Author	Aim of study	Design	Sensitivity	Specificity
Amirfeyz et al (2005)	To investigate the sensitivity and specificity of the hand elevation test, Phalen's test and Tinel's test	Correlation of 46 subjects' hand elevation test findings with post-surgical outcome findings	88%	98%

FINKELSTEIN TEST

The Finkelstein test is designed to test for tenosynovitis of abductor pollicis longus and the extensor pollicis brevis tendons (De Quervain's). The procedure of the test involves the clinician applying a stretch to the structures involved by positioning the thumb into the patient's grip and adding ulnar deviation. The resultant stretch acts to induce a traction force to the tendons, which may elicit the patient's symptoms. An expected positive response from this test is the reproduction of the patient's pain/symptoms over the tested area.

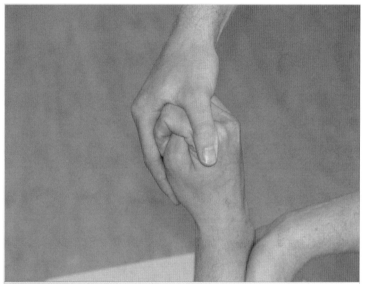

Fig 4.15   Finkelstein test. The patient grasps their own thumb in their fist.

PROCEDURE
Patient: The patient is positioned in sitting. Their thumb is positioned in opposition across their palm. The patient grasps their thumb with their fingers (Fig. 4.15).
Clinician: The clinician stands alongside the patient, passively adding ulnar deviation to the wrist (Fig. 4.16).

FINDINGS
Positive result: Pain reported over the radial styloid process may indicate De Quervian's tenosynovitis.
Negative result: There is no pain or reproduction of symptoms reported by the patient.

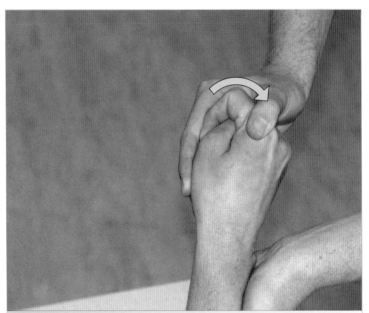

Fig 4.16 Finkelstein test. The clinician applies ulnar deviation and assesses for symptom reproduction over the radial styloid.

JERSEY FINGER SIGN

The Jersey finger sign is designed to test for a rupture of the flexor digitorum profundus tendon at the distal interphalangeal joint. This test is also known as 'sweater finger sign'. The procedure of the test involves asking the patient to form a fist and flex their fingers into their palm. If a rupture of the flexor digitorum profundus tendon at the distal interphalangeal joint has occurred the patient will be unable to flex the affected finger at the distal interphalangeal joint fully into their palm. Jersey finger often occurs during contact sports, where the patient has tried to grab an opponent's jersey and has caught their finger; it most commonly occurs at the ring finger. The distal interphalangeal joint is momentarily hyperextended and results in a flexor digitorum profundus tendon rupture. An expected positive response from this test is the inability of the patient to flex their affected finger into the palm.

PROCEDURE

Patient: The patient is positioned in sitting and attempts to make a fist with the affected hand (Fig. 4.17).

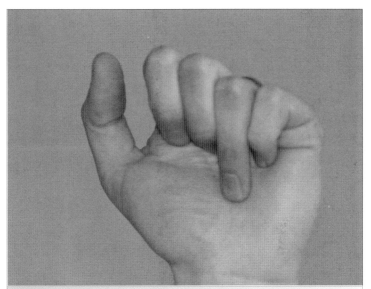

Fig 4.17   Jersey finger sign. Failure to flex the distal interphalangeal joint may indicate a rupture of the flexor digitorum profundus tendon.

Clinician: The clinician stands alongside the patient and assesses whether the patient can fully flex all the distal interphalangeal joints.

FINDINGS

Positive result: A failure of the distal interphalangeal joint to flex, resulting in the tip of the finger failing to form the fist position on the affected finger, may suggest a rupture of flexor digitorum profundus tendon at the distal interphalangeal joint.

Negative result: The patient can form a fist with all their fingers.

FROMENT'S SIGN

Froment's sign is designed to test the integrity of the ulnar nerve. The procedure of the test involves the patient forming a pinch grip with their index finger and thumb (Fig. 4.18). Failure to maintain the contact, with the distal phalangeal joint of the index finger extending, may indicate an ulnar nerve lesion. Froment's sign is identical to the pinch grip test. The reason for this is that the pinch grip action is supplied by both the median and ulnar nerves. Damage to the ulnar nerve can lead to specific muscle power loss of adductor pollicis and the interossei muscles, depending upon the site of the lesion. An expected positive response from this test is the inability to maintain a pinch grip.

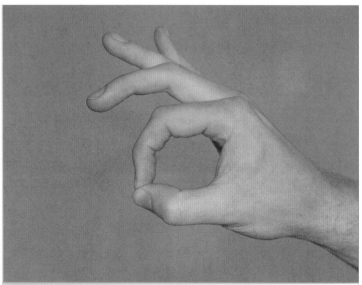

Fig 4.18   Froment's sign. The patient attempts to form a pinch grip between their thumb and index finger.

PROCEDURE

Patient: The patient is positioned in sitting or standing and attempts to make a pinch grip with their thumb and index finger.
Clinician: The clinician is positioned alongside the patient and instructs the patient to form a pinch grip, between their thumb and index finger.

FINDINGS

Positive result: The patient is unable to form a tip-to-tip link between the thumb and index finger, with an inability to prevent the distal interphalangeal joint from extending, leading to a pad-to-pad contact of the thumb and finger rather than a tip-to-tip contact (Fig. 4.19).
Negative result: There is a firm grip between the thumb and index finger.

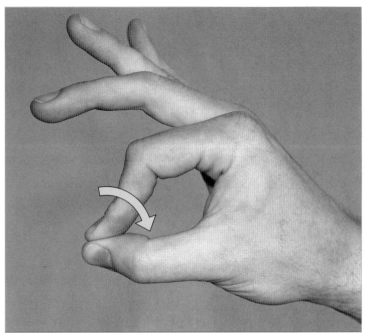

Fig 4.19   Froment's sign. Failure to maintain a tip-to-tip contact indicates a positive result.

REFERENCES

Amirfeyz R, Gozzard C, Leslie I 2005 Hand elevation test for assessment of carpal tunnel syndrome. Journal of Hand Surgery 30(4): 361–364

Brüske J, Bednarski M, Grzelec H et al 2002 The usefulness of the Phalen test and the Hoffmann–Tinel sign in the diagnosis of carpal tunnel syndrome. Acta Orthopaedica Belgica 68(2): 141–145

Kuhlman K, Hennessey W 1997 Sensitivity and specificity of carpal tunnel syndrome signs. American Journal of Physical Medicine and Rehabilitation 76(6): 451–457

LaJoie A, McCabe S, Thomas B et al 2005 Determining the sensitivity and specificity of common diagnostic tests for carpal tunnel syndrome using latent class analysis. Plastic and Reconstructive Surgery 116(2): 502–507

MacDermid J, Wessel J 2004 Clinical diagnosis of carpal tunnel: a systematic review. Journal of Hand Therapy 17(2): 309–319

Massy-Westropp N, Grimmer K, Bain G 2000 A systematic review of the clinical diagnostic tests for carpal tunnel syndrome. Journal of Hand Surgery 25(1): 120–127

Tetro A, Evanoff B, Hollstien S et al 1998 A new provocative test for carpal tunnel syndrome. Journal of Bone and Joint Surgery 80(3): 493–498

BIBLIOGRAPHY AND FURTHER READING

Forman T, Forman S, Nicholas R 2005 A clinical approach to diagnosing wrist pain. American Family Physician 72(9): 1753–1758

Magee D 2008 Orthopedic physical assessment, 5th edn. Saunders Elsevier, St Louis, MO

Nakamura R, Horii E, Imaeda T et al 1997 The ulnocarpal stress test in the diagnosis of ulnar-sided wrist pain. Journal of Hand Surgery 2(6): 719–723

Norris C 2005 Sports injuries diagnosis and management, 3rd edn. Butterworth-Heinemann, Edinburgh

Richardson C, Faber G 2003 Froment's sign. Journal of Visual Communication in Medicine 26(1): 34

The pelvis

ANTERIOR GAPPING TEST

The anterior gapping test is designed to identify whether pain is arising from the sacroiliac joint. This test is also known as the 'distraction test'. The procedure of the test involves the clinician applying a gapping or distraction force to the anterior aspect of the pelvis by pushing the anterior superior iliac spines away from each other. This action results in a potential compression force transmitted to the posterior aspect of the pelvis. Compression of the articular surfaces of the sacroiliac joint may result in compression of sensitized musculoskeletal structures. An expected positive response from this test is the reproduction of the patient's pain or symptoms.

PROCEDURE
Patient: The patient is positioned in supine on a plinth.
Clinician: The clinician stands alongside the patient, with their right and left hands positioned so that the palm pushes against the medial aspect of the anterior superior iliac spines. The clinician applies a horizontal force, attempting to separate the anterior superior iliac spines (Fig. 5.1).

FINDINGS
Positive result: The production of pain, normally located around the sacroiliac joint, may indicate that the application of

force during the test procedure has sensitized or put pressure through damaged structures within or around the sacroiliac joint. It is possible that reproduction of symptoms for the patient in areas commonly referred to by the sacroiliac joint may also indicate a positive result.

Negative result: No reproduction of pain.

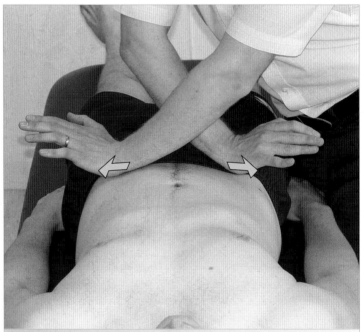

Fig 5.1   Anterior gapping test. The clinician applies a gapping force to the anterior superior iliac spines, which results in a compressive force being transmitted to the sacroiliac joint and monitors for reproduction of symptoms.

Table 5.1 Sensitivity and specificity values of the anterior gapping test

Author	Aim of study	Design	Sensitivity	Specificity
van der Wurff et al (2000)	Review the validity of sacroiliac joint pain provocation and mobility tests	Systematic review of four studies that met the selection criteria	Range 11–21%	Range 90–100%

ANTERIOR COMPRESSION TEST

The anterior compression test is designed to identify whether pain is arising from the sacroiliac joint. This test is also known as the 'compression test'. The procedure of the test involves the clinician applying a compression force to the anterior aspect of the pelvis by pushing the anterior superior iliac spines towards each other. This action results in a potential distraction force transmitted to the posterior aspect of the pelvis. Distraction of the articular surfaces of the sacroiliac joint may result in distraction of sensitized musculoskeletal structures. An expected positive response from this test is the reproduction of the patient's pain or symptoms.

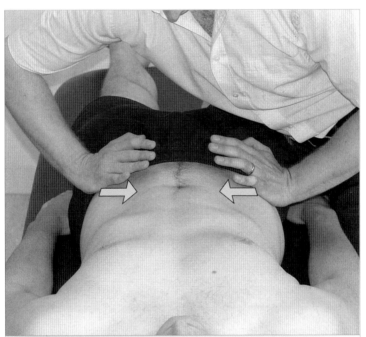

Fig 5.2   Anterior compression test. The clinician applies a compression force to the anterior superior iliac spines, which results in a distraction force being transmitted to the sacroiliac joint, and monitors for reproduction of symptoms.

PROCEDURE
  Patient: The patient is positioned in supine on a plinth.
  Clinician: The clinician stands alongside the patient, applying a compression force to the lateral aspect of the anterior part of the

pelvis adjacent to the anterior superior iliac spines. The palms of the hands are situated on the lateral aspects of the anterior superior iliac spines. The clinician applies a horizontal force to compress the two pelvic bones (Fig. 5.2).

FINDINGS

Positive result: The production of pain, normally located around the sacroiliac joint, may indicate that the application of force during the test procedure has sensitized or applied a stretch force through damaged structures round the sacroiliac joint. It is possible that reproduction of symptoms for the patient in areas commonly referred to by the sacroiliac joint may also indicate a positive result.

Negative result: No reproduction of pain.

Table 5.2 Sensitivity and specificity values of the anterior compression test

Author	Aim of study	Design	Sensitivity	Specificity
van der Wurff et al (2000)	Review the validity of sacroiliac joint pain provocation and mobility tests	Systematic review of four studies that met the selection criteria	Range 0–19%	Range 90–100%

GAENSLEN'S TEST

Gaenslen's test is designed to identify whether pain is arising from the sacroiliac joint. This test is also known as 'Gaenslen's manoeuvre'. The procedure of the test involves applying either a posterior or anterior rotational force through the sacroiliac joint in a weight-bearing position. This rotational force acts to load sensitized musculoskeletal structures within and adjacent to the sacroiliac joint. An expected positive response from this test is the reproduction of the patient's pain or symptoms.

PROCEDURE

Patient: The patient is positioned in supine on the edge of a plinth, one leg hanging over the edge, producing hip extension,

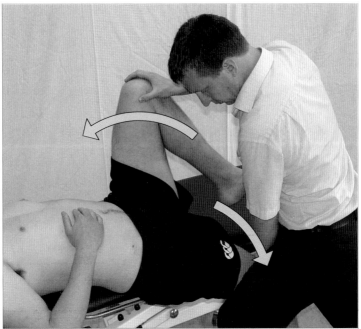

Fig 5.3 Gaenslen's test. The clinician produces a torsion force to the sacroiliac joint by applying flexion of one hip and extension of the other, and monitors for reproduction of symptoms.

and the other hip and knee flexed up to the chest with the patient holding onto the knee with both hands.

Clinician: The clinician stands alongside the plinth and applies an opposing force to each leg thus encouraging the rotational force through the sacroiliac joint (Fig. 5.3).

FINDINGS

Positive result: Production of pain or reproduction of the patient's symptoms may indicate that the torsion effect has put stress on to the soft tissue structure of the sacroiliac joint, thus generating the patient's pain. It is possible that reproduction of symptoms for the patient in areas commonly referred to by the sacroiliac joint may also indicate a positive result.

Negative result: No reproduction of pain.

Table 5.3 Sensitivity and specificity values of Gaenslen's test

Author	Aim of study	Design	Sensitivity	Specificity
Kokmeyer et al (2002)	To assess the inter-rater reliability of five common sacroiliac joint pain provocation tests. Also included a mini analysis of the sensitivity and specificity literature	Review of the available literature. Identified one study investigating the sensitivity and specificity of Gaenslen's test	Range 56–86%	Range 11–40%
van der Wurff et al (2000)	Review the validity of sacroiliac joint pain provocation and mobility tests	Systematic review of three studies that met the selection criteria	Range 21–71%	Range 26–72%

THIGH THRUST TEST

The thigh thrust test is designed to identify whether pain is arising from the sacroiliac joint. The procedure involves placing the patient's hip into 90° of flexion and applying a force directly down through the line of the femur so that it produces a shearing force through the sacroiliac joint. To stop the plinth reducing the application of the force the clinician positions their hand on to the sacral base, enabling a small range of movement of the ilium on the sacrum to take place. This test may lead to the stressing of soft tissue or bony structures that may be responsible for the patient's pain. An expected positive response from this test is the reproduction of the patient's pain or symptoms.

PROCEDURE

Patient: The patient is positioned in supine on a plinth. The leg to be tested should have: hip 90°, knee 90° or greater.

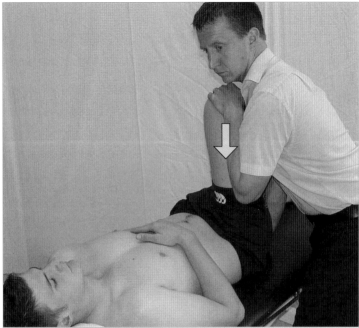

Fig 5.4 Thigh thrust test. The clinician applies a shear force through the sacroiliac joint transmitted via a longitudinal force through the femur, and monitors for reproduction of symptoms.

Clinician: The clinician should be standing alongside the patient, hand positioned under the patient so that it rests between the patient's sacrum and the plinth. The other arm/hand cradles the flexed knee, enabling the transmission of a vertical force down the line of the femur (Fig. 5.4).

FINDINGS

Positive result: Production of pain or reproduction of the patient's symptoms may indicate that the torsion effect has put stress on to the soft tissue structure of the sacroiliac joint, thus generating pain. It is possible that reproduction of symptoms for the patient in areas commonly referred to by the sacroiliac joint may also indicate a positive result.

Negative result: No reproduction of pain.

Table 5.4 Sensitivity and specificity values of the thigh thrust test

Author	Aim of study	Design	Sensitivity	Specificity
Kokmeyer et al (2002)	To assess the inter-rater reliability of five common sacroiliac joint pain provocation tests. Also included a mini analysis of the sensitivity and specificity literature	Review of the available literature. Identified three studies investigating the sensitivity and specificity of the thigh thrust test	Range 8–96%	Range 33–92%
van der Wurff et al (2000)	Review the validity of sacroiliac joint pain provocation and mobility tests.	Systematic review of three studies that met the selection criteria	Range 36–80%	Range 50–100%

SHEAR TEST

The shear test is designed to identify whether pain is arising from the sacroiliac joint. This test is also known as the 'sacral thrust technique'. The procedure involves applying a posterior to anterior force through the sacrum while the patient is positioned in prone lying. This action results in the application of a shearing force between the ilium and the sacral articular surfaces. This action may lead to the stressing of soft tissue or bony structures that may be responsible for the patient's pain. An expected positive response from this test is the reproduction of the patient's pain or symptoms.

PROCEDURE
Patient: The patient is positioned in prone on a plinth.
Clinician: The clinician identifies the sacral base by following the iliac crests posteriorly. The clinician then applies a downwards force to the sacrum as close to the sacroiliac joint line as possible (Fig. 5.5).

FINDINGS
Positive result: Production of pain or reproduction of the patient's symptoms may indicate that the torsion effect has put stress on to the soft tissue structures of the sacroiliac joint and thus resulted in generation of the patient's pain. It is possible that reproduction of symptoms

for the patient in areas commonly referred to by the sacroiliac joint may also indicate a positive result.

Negative result: No reproduction of pain.

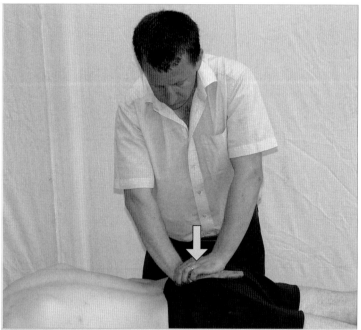

Fig 5.5   Shear test. The clinician applies a shear force to the sacroiliac joint by directly loading the sacrum, and monitors for reproduction of symptoms.

Table 5.5 Sensitivity and specificity values of the shear test

Author	Aim of study	Design	Sensitivity	Specificity
Kokmeyer et al (2002)	To assess the inter-rater reliability of five common sacroiliac joint pain provocation tests. Also included a mini analysis of the sensitivity and specificity literature	Review of the available literature. Identified two studies investigating the sensitivity and specificity of the shear test	Range 19–70%	Range 11–77%
van der Wurff et al (2000)	Review the validity of sacroiliac joint pain provocation and mobility tests	Systematic review of four studies that met the selection criteria	Range 3–53%	Range 29–100%

GILLET'S TEST

Gillet's test is designed to assess the movement available at the sacroiliac joint. This test is also known as the 'stork test'. The procedure of the test involves asking the patient to pull one knee up to their chest while in a standing position. During this movement the clinician assesses for a difference in the quality and available movement from one sacroiliac joint to the other by monitoring the movement of the posterior superior iliac spines. An expected positive result of this test may be identified if there is a restriction or an increase in the movement on the affected side. These findings may indicate that there is, respectively, either a hypomobility or a hypermobility issue of the sacroiliac joint.

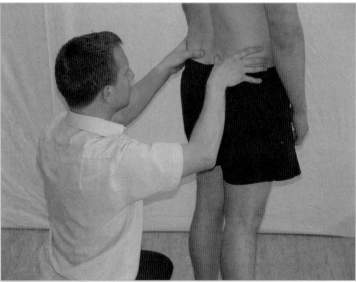

Fig 5.6 Gillet's test. The clinician identifies the patient's posterior superior iliac spines and asks the patient to flex their hip.

PROCEDURE

Patient: The patient is positioned in a standing posture, with their feet shoulder-width apart to establish a stable starting position (Fig. 5.6). The patient could also stabilize themselves by lightly holding on to a raised plinth if necessary.

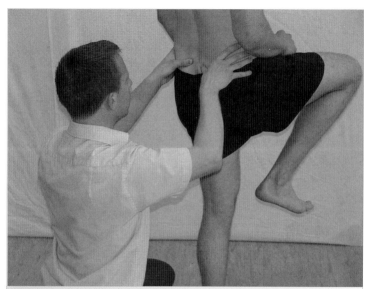

Fig 5.7   Gillet's test. The clinician assesses for differences in the movement of the posterior superior iliac spines from one side to the other.

Clinician: The clinician is positioned seated or crouched behind the patient, with thumbs over the left and right posterior superior iliac spine. The clinician asks the patient to flex a hip to 90° and traces the movement of the thumbs following the posterior superior iliac spines (Fig. 5.7).

FINDINGS

Positive result: An increased movement of the posterior superior iliac spine on the affected sacroiliac joint side may suggest a hypermobility problem in that sacroiliac joint and likewise a decrease in movement on the affected side may suggest a hypomobility problem.

Negative result: Symmetrical movements of the affected side, compared to the non-affected side.

STANDING FLEXION TEST

The standing flexion test is designed to assess the movement available at the sacroiliac joint. This test is also known as the 'forward flexion test' or the 'overtake phenomenon'. The procedure of the test involves asking the patient to bend forward into lumbar flexion from a standing posture with their knees remaining in extension. The clinician assesses for a difference in the quality and available movement from one sacroiliac joint to the other by monitoring the movement of the posterior superior iliac spines. An expected positive result of this test may be identified if there is a restriction or an increase in the movement on the affected side. These findings may indicate that there is, respectively, either a hypomobility or a hypermobility issue of the sacroiliac joint.

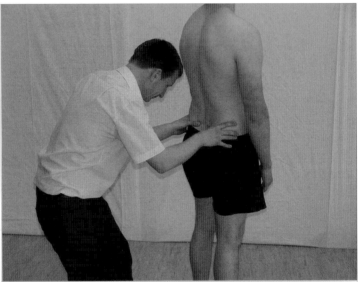

Fig 5.8 Standing flexion test. The clinician identifies the patient's posterior superior iliac spines and asks the patient to bend forward into lumbar flexion.

PROCEDURE

Patient: The patient is positioned in a standing posture, with their feet shoulder-width apart to establish a stable starting position (Fig. 5.8).

Clinician: The clinician is positioned behind the patient with both thumbs on the posterior superior iliac spine. The clinician asks the patient to bend forwards while keeping the knees extended, and monitors the movement of the posterior superior iliac spines in relation to each other (Fig. 5.9).

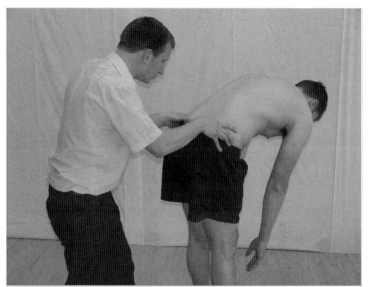

Fig 5.9   Standing flexion test. The clinician assesses for differences in the movement of the posterior superior iliac spines from one side to the other.

FINDINGS

Positive result: An increased movement of the posterior superior iliac spine on the affected sacroiliac joint side may suggest a hypermobility problem in that sacroiliac joint and likewise a decrease in movement on the affected side may suggest a hypomobility problem.

Negative result: Symmetrical movements of the affected side, compared to the non-affected side.

SEATED FLEXION TEST

The seated flexion test is designed to assess the movement available at the sacroiliac joint. The procedure of the test involves asking the patient to bend forwards into lumbar flexion in a seated posture with their feet flat on the floor. The clinician assesses for any difference in the quality and available movement from one sacroiliac joint to the other by monitoring the movement of the posterior superior iliac spines. An expected positive result of this test may be identified if there is a restriction or an increase in the movement on the affected side. These findings may indicate, respectively, that there is either a hypomobility or a hypermobility issue of the sacroiliac joint.

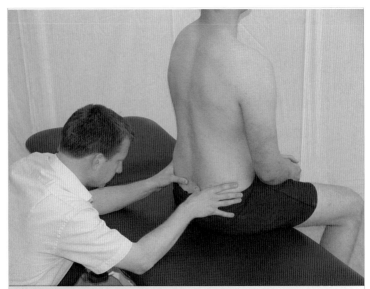

Fig 5.10 Seated flexion test. The clinician identifies the patient's posterior superior iliac spines and asks the patient to bend forward into lumbar flexion.

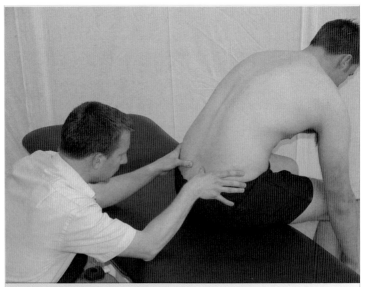

Fig 5.11 Seated flexion test. The clinician assesses for differences in the movement of the posterior superior iliac spines from one side to the other.

PROCEDURE

Patient: The patient is seated on the edge of a plinth with their hips and knees in 90° flexion. The patient's feet are flat on the floor (Fig. 5.10).

Clinician: The clinician is positioned behind the patient with both thumbs on the posterior superior iliac spine. The clinician asks the patient to bend forwards and take their hands down to the floor, which prevents the patient altering the position by using the upper limbs to redistribute their upper body weight. The clinician monitors the movement of the posterior superior iliac spines in relation to each other (Fig. 5.11).

FINDINGS

Positive result: An increased movement of the posterior superior iliac spine on the affected sacroiliac joint side may suggest a hypermobility problem in that sacroiliac joint and likewise a decrease in movement on the affected side may suggest a hypomobility problem.

Negative result: Symmetrical movements of the affected side, compared to the non-affected side.

PATRICK'S SIGN

Patrick's sign is designed to identify whether pain is arising from the sacroiliac joint, the hip joint or the lumbar spine. This test is also known as the 'FABER test'. The procedure of the test involves positioning the hip joint into flexion, abduction and external rotation; this action may identify whether pain is arising from the hip joint or the sacroiliac joint. This position loads the hip joint and in turn may result in a force being transmitted through to the sacroiliac joint. If pain is elicited then the lumbar spine may be a less likely cause of the patient's symptoms. The term FABER is a useful mnemonic, which acts as a reminder as to the end position of the hip joint for the test: Flexion, ABduction, External Rotation. Within the literature there are differences in the application of the test; furthermore, there are also differences regarding interpretation of test findings.

PROCEDURE

Patient: The patient is positioned in supine on a plinth, with the knee flexed to approximately 90° and the hip in the F.AB. ER. position of flexion, abduction and external rotation. The patient's foot is resting on the opposite knee.

Clinician: The clinician assists the patient in adopting the position by moving the leg passively. The clinician then assesses for a difference in the range of movement from the affected side to the non-affected side and notes any potential symptom reproduced during the test. The clinician may also add overpressure to the movement (Figs 5.12 and 5.13).

FINDINGS

Positive result: A decrease in the range of movement, signified by the amount the knee drops towards the plinth, may suggest hip joint or sacroiliac joint pathology or muscle tightness around the hip joint. Additional overpressure may also provide information as to the end feel of the combination movement. Pain on either patient position or on clinician applied overpressure may be indicative of hip joint, sacroiliac joint or muscular pathology when compared to the non-affected side. Indication of any of the above may indicate that pain or loss of range is occurring due to a dysfunction in either the hip or sacroiliac joint or the soft tissues surrounding these areas. A positive finding may also imply that the symptoms are not arising from the lumbar spine specifically.

Negative result: No change in range or end feel on either of the test procedures and/or no reproduction of symptoms may suggest no involvement of the implied structures.

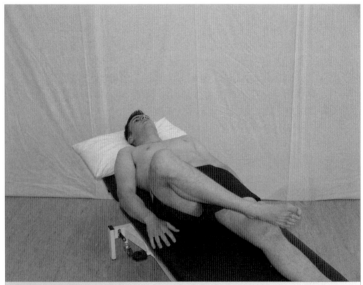

Fig 5.12 Patrick's sign. The patient adopts the position of flexion, abduction and external rotation of the hip joint. The clinician assesses for symptom reproduction and potential loss of range of movement.

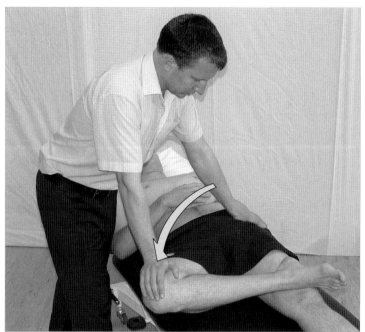

Fig 5.13 Patrick's sign. The clinician may apply overpressure to assess the end feel of the combination movement and monitor symptom reproduction.

Table 5.6 Sensitivity and specificity values of Patrick's sign

Author	Aim of study	Design	Sensitivity	Specificity
Kokmeyer et al (2002)	To assess the inter-rater reliability of five common sacroiliac joint pain provocation tests. Also included an analysis of the sensitivity and specificity literature	Review of the available literature. Identified two studies investigating the sensitivity and specificity of Patrick's sign	Range 1–84%	Range 4–99%
van der Wurff et al (2000)	Review the validity of sacroiliac joint pain provocation and mobility tests	Systematic review of four studies that met the selection criteria	Range 57–77%	Range 16–100%

REFERENCES

Kokmeyer D, van der Wurff P, Aufdemkampe G et al 2002 The reliability of multitest regimens with sacroiliac pain provocation tests. Journal of Manipulative Physiological Therapy 25(1): 42–48

van der Wurff P, Meyne W, Hagmeijer R 2000 Clinical tests of the sacroiliac joint: a systematic methodological review part 2: Validity. Manual Therapy 5(2): 89–96

BIBLIOGRAPHY AND FURTHER READING

Laslett M, Young S, Aprill C et al 2003 Diagnosing painful sacroiliac joints: a validity study of a McKenzie evaluation and sacroiliac provocation tests. Australian Journal of Physiotherapy 49(2): 89–97

Laslett M, Aprill C, McDonald B et al 2005 Diagnosis of sacroiliac joint pain: validity of individual provocation tests and composites of tests. Manual Therapy 10(3): 207–218

Magee D 2008 Orthopedic physical assessment, 5th edn. Saunders Elsevier, St Louis, MO

Norris C 2005 Sports injuries diagnosis and management, 3rd edn. Butterworth-Heinemann, Edinburgh

Riddle D, Freburger J 2002 Evaluation of the presence of sacroiliac joint region dysfunction using a combination of tests: a multicenter intertester reliability study. Physical Therapy 82(8): 772–781

van der Wurff P, Hagmeijer R, Meyne W 2000 Clinical tests of the sacroiliac joint: a systematic methodological review part 1: Reliability. Manual Therapy 5(1): 30–36

The hip

TRENDELENBURG TEST

The Trendelenburg test is designed to test for muscle weakness or instability around the hip joint. The procedure of the test involves the clinician asking the patient to stand on the affected leg. If there is weakness of the stabilizing muscles around the hip joint the hip will drop out and backwards. The main muscle group affected is often the glutei, which have a key role in maintaining single leg balance as well as in the stance phase during gait. An expected positive response from this test is a visual dropping out of the hip in a posterolateral direction.

PROCEDURE

Patient: The patient is positioned in a standing posture, with their feet shoulder-width apart to establish a stable starting position. The patient could also stabilize themselves by lightly holding on to a raised plinth if necessary (Fig. 6.1).

Clinician: The clinician asks the patient to lift their non-affected foot off the floor by flexing their hip. The clinician observes for any identified movements of the pelvis and hips.

FINDINGS

Positive result: The affected hip drops laterally or posterolaterally, often with a sudden release, as if giving way (Fig. 6.2).

Negative result: There is no evidence of giving way of the hip when standing on the affected leg.

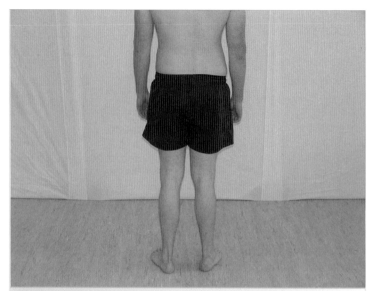

Fig 6.1 Trendelenburg test. The clinician observes the patient from behind and asks them to lift their foot off the floor.

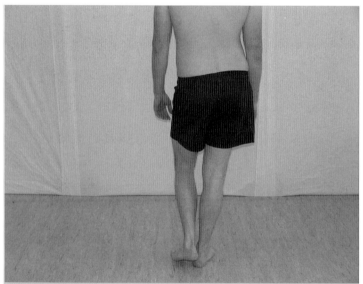

Fig 6.2 Trendelenburg test. A dropping out of the hip indicates a positive result.

OBER'S TEST

Ober's test is designed to test for tightness in the iliotibial tract. The procedure of the test involves positioning the patient into side lying as a way of optimizing the available stretch of the iliotibial tract. Applying a stretch to the iliotibial tract enables the clinician to assess for a difference in the available range of the hip joint, compared to the non-affected leg. An expected positive response from this test is the identification of tightness in the iliotibial tract on the affected side. The test may also reproduce the patient's symptoms.

PROCEDURE

Patient: The patient is positioned in side lying on a plinth, with the side to be tested uppermost. The hip and knee of the lower leg are positioned in 90° flexion; this produces enough space to allow the upper leg to drop down towards the plinth. The uppermost leg position is knee extended, hip positioned into 10–20° of extension (Fig. 6.3).

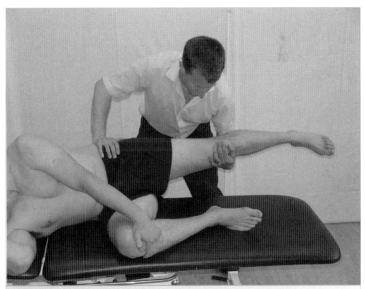

Fig 6.3 Ober's test. The clinician supports the patient's pelvis and supports the patient's leg at the knee joint.

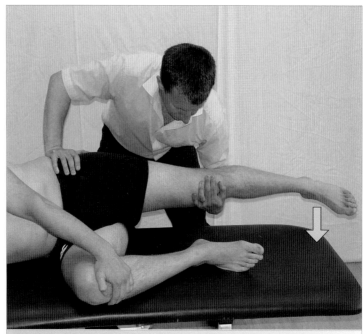

Fig 6.4 Ober's test. The clinician slowly drops the leg towards the plinth and assesses the available range of adduction and notes any symptom reproduction.

Clinician: The clinician stabilizes the pelvis to ensure no trick movement occurs. The clinician supports the uppermost leg and lowers the leg towards the plinth (Fig. 6.4).

FINDINGS
Positive result: If the affected hip fails to drop as far towards the plinth as the non-affected hip this may suggest iliotibial tract tightness. The test may also reproduce the patient's symptoms.
Negative result: An equal range of movement of both the affected and non-affected hip, with no reproduction of the patient's symptoms.

THE THOMAS TEST

The Thomas test is designed to differentiate between tightness of the hip flexors and rectus femoris. The procedure of the test involves positioning the patient so the lumbar spine and pelvis are fixed, from where the additional flexion or extension of the knee joint can differentiate between iliopsoas or rectus femoris. Due to the action of the bi-articular muscle, flexion of the knee may lead to flexion of the hip where there is rectus femoris tightness, whereas a lack of hip flexion during knee flexion may indicate tightness of iliopsoas. The clinician can then assess the difference between the affected and non-affected side. An expected positive response from this test is the identification of tightness in either the independent hip flexors or rectus femoris. The test may also reproduce the patient's symptoms.

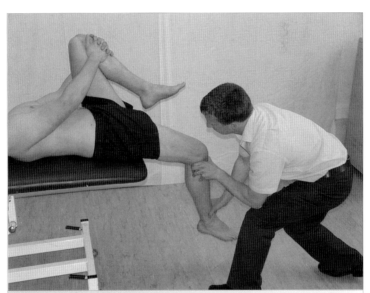

Fig 6.5 The Thomas test. The patient is positioned on the end of the plinth, holding one knee to the chest and letting the other leg hang down with gravity.

PROCEDURE

Patient: The patient is positioned in supine on a plinth, towards the bottom of the plinth, to allow the lower leg to hang off the end. The patient is instructed to hold the non-affected leg to the chest with both arms. This acts to pull the pelvis into posterior rotation and as the patient is lying down the weight of the affected leg is pulled down with gravity (Fig. 6.5).

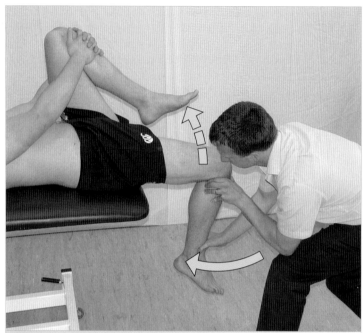

Fig 6.6 The Thomas test. The clinician applies knee flexion and observes for flexion occurring at the hip joint.

Clinician: The clinician supports the patient's position and assesses the movement of the affected side by passively flexing the patient's knee. The test is then repeated on the opposite side and any difference in range or symptom reproduction is noted (Fig. 6.6).

FINDINGS

Positive result: A lack of hip extension in either position of knee flexion or extension may suggest tightness in either rectus femoris or iliopsoas. If the hip flexes during knee flexion, this may suggest that rectus femoris is the leading cause of the limitation of range, but if the hip fails to flex as the knee is flexed, this may suggest that iliopsoas is responsible for the limitation of range. The test may also reproduce the patient's symptoms.

Negative results: There will be no change in the range or symptoms during testing. It should be noted there is no 'normal' for this test and some subjects may demonstrate rectus femoris tightness and others may demonstrate iliopsoas tightness; however, what is to be noted is if there is a difference between the affected and the non-affected side.

ELY TEST

The Ely test is designed to test for a contracture or spasticity of rectus femoris. This test is also known as the 'Duncan–Ely test'. The procedure of the test involves a rapid flexion of the knee by the clinician while the patient is positioned in prone. The rapid lengthening of rectus femoris may elicit signs of spasticity. The Ely test is more commonly used within the neurology specialty, to identify potential neurological changes in muscle tone. However, it may be used within the musculoskeletal specialty to try and determine a possible cause of loss of hip extension. An expected positive response from this test is the identification of possible neurological abnormalities in muscle tone, and potential loss of hip extension.

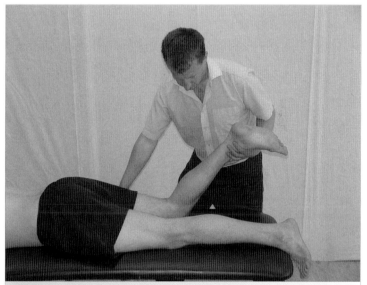

Fig 6.7   Ely test. The patient is positioned prone on the plinth; the clinician ensures that the muscles to be tested are relaxed.

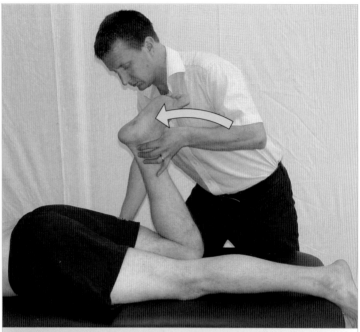

Fig 6.8 Ely test. The clinician applies rapid knee flexion and monitors for any resistance during the movement.

PROCEDURE
Patient: The patient is positioned prone on a plinth (Fig. 6.7).
Clinician: The clinician gently grasps the patient's foot and rapidly flexes the knee so that the foot moves towards the buttock (Fig. 6.8).

FINDINGS
Positive result: A resistance or catching within the mid-range of the movement together with a decreased range of movement may suggest a rectus femoris contracture. The clinician may also note a rising up of the patient's pelvis off the plinth, which may indicate hip flexor tightness.
Negative result: The knee flexes to its full range and the pelvis remains in the starting position.

FULCRUM TEST

The fulcrum test is designed to identify a potential stress fracture of the femur. The procedure of the test involves loading the hip joint by pushing the head of the femur up into the acetabulum. The clinician's hand, positioned under the patient's thigh, acts as a fulcrum and further loads the shaft of the femur. The clinician can reposition their hand under the thigh to create various points of loading along the femoral shaft. This may be useful if the symptoms are difficult to elicit. Within the field of musculoskeletal assessment it is rare that fractures are missed in the initial triage process. However, a stress fracture can be difficult to identify as it is not normally associated with immediate trauma. An expected positive response from this test is the reproduction of the patient's pain or symptoms.

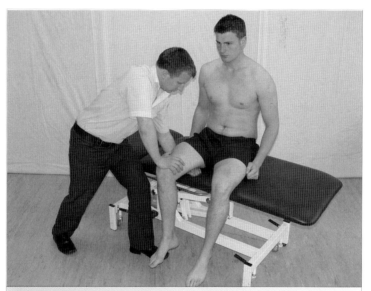

Fig 6.9 Fulcrum test. The clinician places their hand under the shaft of the femur to act as a fulcrum.

PROCEDURE

Patient: The patient is positioned in sitting on a plinth, legs hanging over the edge, feet just off the floor (Fig. 6.9).

Clinician: The clinician is positioned alongside the patient with one hand under the mid-part of their thigh. The other hand applies a downwards pressure to the knee joint. The clinician then compares the affected side to the non-affected side (Fig. 6.10).

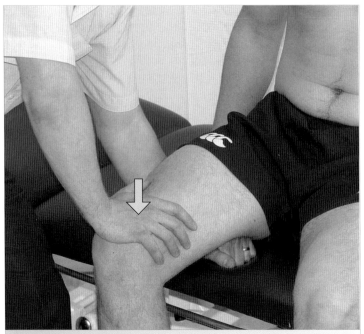

Fig 6.10 Fulcrum test. The clinician applies a force through the distal end of the femur, loading the hip joint, and monitors for symptom reproduction.

FINDINGS

Positive result: Acute bony-type pain, along the femoral shaft or located within the patient's groin, in the vicinity of the hip joint line, may suggest a stress fracture of the femur.

Negative result: No production of pain along the femoral shaft or in the patient's groin.

HOP TEST

The hop test is designed to identify a potential stress fracture of the femur. The procedure of the test involves loading the hip joint and the femur by asking the patient to perform a hop on the affected leg. The loading of the hip joint and femur occurs as the patient lands from the hop activity. The force of impact is transmitted through the femur and may well act to elicit pain over a stress fracture site. Caution should be paramount when applying this test, as the test procedure may itself induce pain inhibition and could lead to a fall. The test should be performed in a suitable environment to prevent risk of falls. An expected positive response from this test is the production of pain over a stress fracture site on impact from the hop activity. Furthermore, the stress fracture may act to inhibit the patient's ability to perform the activity.

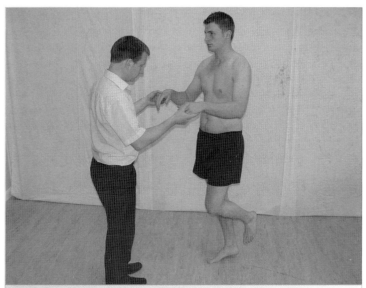

Fig 6.11   Hop test. The clinician stabilizes the patient and asks them to hop on the non-affected leg then on the affected leg, and assesses for ability and symptom reproduction.

PROCEDURE

Patient: The patient is asked to hop on the non-affected leg first so that the clinician can assess the patient's normal ability.

Clinician: The clinician should remain close to the patient to provide any necessary support or assistance. Also, the clinician should request that the patient attempts one hop on each leg first. The repetition could then be increased, as gauged by the patient's ability (Fig. 6.11).

FINDINGS

Positive result: An acute bony pain normally elicited on the first or second hop may suggest a stress fracture over the site of pain. The patient may also describe or demonstrate a lack of ability to perform the task; this may also suggest a substantial pathology, such as a stress fracture. Any suspicion of a bony injury should be referred for appropriate medical investigation as physiotherapeutic interventions may be contraindicated.

Negative result: A patient who performs a hop with no pain may not have a stress fracture. Similarly, a patient who can hop multiple times (for example, 10 repetitions) may also not be suffering from a stress fracture, as this level of ability does not correlate with the usual presentation of a stress fracture.

BIBLIOGRAPHY AND FURTHER READING

Magee D 2008 Orthopedic physical assessment, 5th edn. Saunders Elsevier, St Louis, MO

Marks M, Alexander J, Sutherland D et al 2003 Clinical utility of the Duncan–Ely test for rectus femoris dysfunction during the swing phase of gait. Developmental Medicine and Child Neurology 45(11): 763–768

Mitchell B, McCrory P, Brukner P et al 2003 Hip joint pathology: clinical presentation and correlation between magnetic resonance arthrography, ultrasound and arthroscopic findings in 25 consecutive cases. Clinical Journal of Sports Medicine 13(3): 152–156

Norris C 2005 Sports injuries diagnosis and management, 3rd edn. Butterworth-Heinemann, Edinburgh

Peeler J, Anderson J 2007 Reliability of the Thomas test for assessing range of motion about the hip. Physical Therapy in Sport 8(1): 14–21

The knee

SWEEP TEST

The sweep test is designed to test for an effusion or swelling within the knee joint. This test is also known as the 'bulge test' and the 'brush test'. The procedure of the test involves the clinician gently sweeping the palm of their hand along the medial aspect of the patella five or six times. This action pushes any fluid within the knee joint towards the lateral compartment. A single sweep on the lateral side by the clinician acts to push the collected fluid back medially. Even a small amount of extra fluid within the capsule of the knee joint can result in a visual change in the normal external contours of the knee joint. An expected positive response from this test is a visual movement of fluid from the lateral to the medial aspect of the knee joint.

PROCEDURE

Patient: The patient is positioned in long sitting on a plinth with the quadriceps relaxed. The knee is positioned into full, but not forced, extension.

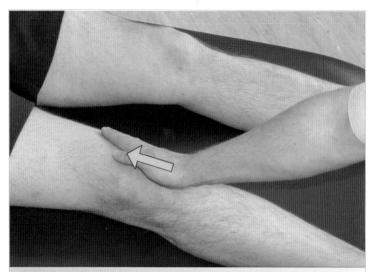

Fig 7.1 Sweep test. The clinician sweeps their hand from distal to proximal on the medial aspect of the patella five or six times.

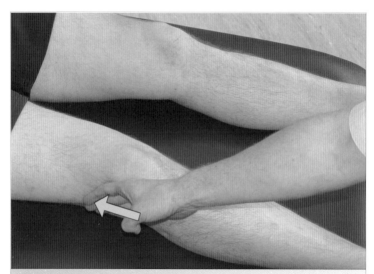

Fig 7.2 Sweep test. The clinician makes a single sweep on the lateral side and observes for movement of fluid towards the medial compartment of the knee joint.

Clinician: The clinician sweeps the palm of their hand from distal to proximal on the medial aspect of the knee joint around the medial edge of the patella (Fig. 7.1). After approximately 5–6 sweeps, make one sweep on the lateral side in a strong distal to proximal motion (Fig. 7.2).

FINDINGS

Positive result: There is a noticeable movement of tissue fluid from the lateral side of the patella to the medial side on the final lateral sweep, suggesting there is a possible effusion present within the knee joint.

Negative result: No noticeable movement of effusion/tissue fluid on the secondary lateral sweep.

PATELLA TAP TEST

The 'patella tap test' is designed to test for an effusion or swelling within the knee joint. The procedure of the test involves the clinician applying a firm but gentle tap to the anterior surface of the patella while the patient's knee is positioned in extension or very slight flexion. If swelling is present within the knee joint the clinician may hear an audible or perceive a palpable 'tap' as the patella hits the anterior surface of the femoral condyles. The excess fluid within the knee joint increases the distance between the femur and the patella, but as the test is performed the force applied by the clinician pushes the excess fluid out of the way and results in the patella being able to tap against the condyles. An expected positive response from this test is an audible or palpable tap as the articular surfaces of the patella make contact with the respective femoral condyles.

PROCEDURE

Patient: The patient is positioned in long sitting on a plinth with the quadriceps relaxed. The knee is positioned in extension or slight flexion.

Clinician: The clinician stabilizes the knee and gently taps the patella against the anterior aspect of the femoral condyles (Fig. 7.3).

FINDINGS

Positive result: There is an audible or palpable 'tap' as the patella hits against the femoral condyles. The presence of a tap may suggest there is excess fluid within the knee joint.

Negative result: No audible or palpable tap may suggest no excess fluid within the knee joint.

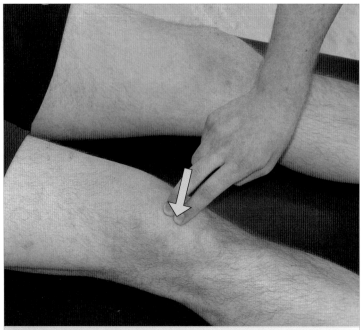

Fig 7.3   Patella tap. The clinician taps the patella against the femoral condyles.

ANTERIOR DRAWER TEST

The anterior drawer test is designed to test for ligament integrity of the anterior cruciate ligament of the knee. The procedure involves the clinician applying a slow, gradual posterior to anterior translation of the tibia while the knee joint is in 90° of flexion. As the anterior translation of the tibia occurs, the anterior cruciate ligament, if intact, should tighten and stop the movement. If the anterior cruciate ligament is ruptured there is no restriction to the anterior glide, thus resulting in an altered end feel of the movement. An expected positive response from this test is an increase in the available anterior translation of the tibia, with a corresponding alteration in the resultant end feel of the movement.

PROCEDURE

Patient: The patient is positioned in long sitting on a plinth. The hip is flexed to approximately 40°, knee flexed to approximately 90°, foot resting on the plinth, ankle in corresponding plantarflexion.

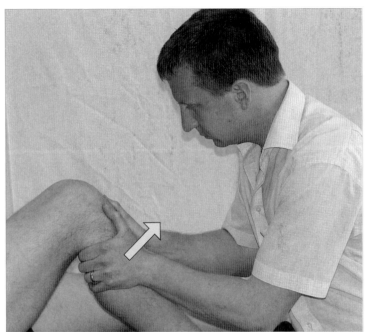

Fig 7.4 Anterior drawer test. The clinician draws the tibia forwards and assesses the available range and end feel of the movement.

Clinician: In practice the clinician often sits on the edge of the plinth and slightly on the patient's foot to stabilize it. The clinician identifies the knee joint line and grasps the superior aspect of the tibia; keeping the thumbs on the joint line either side of the patella tendon, the clinician pulls the tibia forward. Clinically, you may see this test performed as a slow anterior glide of the tibia on the femur, or a quicker jerking movement (Fig. 7.4).

FINDINGS

Positive result: A soft end feel to the anterior translation, or excessive anterior translation compared to the non-affected knee, may suggest that the anterior cruciate ligament has been ruptured.

Negative result: Equal translation of the tibia from the non-affected knee to the affected knee, and a hard end feel to the anterior translation movement.

Table 7.1 Sensitivity and specificity values of the anterior drawer test

Author	Aim of study	Design	Sensitivity	Specificity
Benjaminse et al (2006)	To define the accuracy of clinical tests for assessing anterior cruciate ligament ruptures	Meta-analysis of 28 studies that met selection criteria	Pooled value 92%	Pooled value 91%
Malanga et al (2003)	To present the original descriptions of the common orthopaedic physical examination manoeuvres of the knee and a review of the literature to support the scientific validity of these tests	Meta-analysis of six studies that met the selection criteria	Range 22.2–95.24%	One study reported >97%
Scholten et al (2003)	Summary of the evidence on the accuracy of tests for assessing anterior cruciate ligament ruptures of the knee	Meta-analysis of 17 studies that met the selection criteria	Range 18–92%	Range 78–99%
Solomon et al (2001)	To analyse the accuracy of clinical examination findings for meniscal or ligamentous knee injuries	Meta-analysis of 23 studies that met the selection criteria	Range 9–93%	Range 23–100%

LACHMAN'S TEST

Lachman's test is designed to test for ligament integrity of the anterior cruciate ligament of the knee. The procedure involves the clinician applying a quick posterior to anterior translation of the tibia while the knee joint is in 15–20° of flexion. As the anterior translation of the tibia occurs, the anterior cruciate ligament, if intact, should tighten and stop the movement. If the anterior cruciate ligament is ruptured there is no restriction to the anterior glide, thus resulting in an altered end feel of the move-ment. An expected positive response from this test is an increase in the available anterior translation of the tibia, with a corre-sponding alteration in the resultant end feel of the movement.

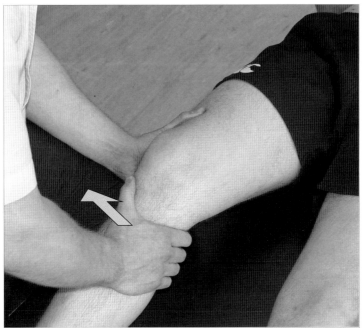

Fig 7.5 Lachman's test. The clinician draws the tibia forwards and assesses the available range and end feel of the movement.

PROCDURE

Patient: The patient is positioned in long sitting on a plinth. Their knee is positioned in 15° of flexion and their foot is resting on the plinth.

Clinician: The clinician stands on the side of the patient to be tested. Clinically, knee flexion is often maintained by resting the patient's knee over the clinician's knee. The clinician's hand is stabilizing the femur and the other hand grasps the calf, below the knee joint line. The clinician must ensure that the patient's hamstrings and quadriceps are relaxed, as they could produce a false positive result. The clinician then initiates a clean forward 'jerk' motion of the hand on the calf, to quickly draw the tibia forwards (Fig. 7.5).

FINDINGS
Positive result: A soft end feel to the anterior translation, or excessive anterior translation compared to the non-affected knee, may suggest that there is a rupture of the anterior cruciate ligament of the knee.

Negative result: Equal translation of the tibia from the non-affected knee to the affected knee, and a hard end feel to the anterior translation movement.

Table 7.2 Sensitivity and specificity values of Lachman's test

Author	Aim of study	Design	Sensitivity	Specificity
Benjaminse et al (2006)	To define the accuracy of clinical tests for assessing anterior cruciate ligament ruptures	Meta-analysis of 28 studies that met selection criteria	Pooled value 85%	Pooled value 94%
Malanga et al (2003)	To present the original descriptions of the common orthopaedic physical examination manoeuvres of the knee and a review of the literature to support the scientific validity of these tests	Meta-analysis of 6 studies that met the selection criteria	Range 80–99%	One study reported 98%
Scholten et al (2003)	Summary of the evidence on the accuracy of tests for assessing anterior cruciate ligament ruptures of the knee	Meta-analysis of 17 studies that met the selection criteria	Range 63–96%	Range 55–100%
Solomon et al (2001)	To analyse the accuracy of clinical examination findings for meniscal or ligamentous knee injuries	Meta-analysis of 23 studies that met the selection criteria	Range 60–100%	100%

PIVOT SHIFT TEST

The pivot shift test is designed to test for ligament integrity of the anterior cruciate ligament of the knee. The procedure involves the clinician applying a medial rotational and a valgus force to the patient's knee, and then slowly extending the knee through its normal range. This combination of forces is thought to result in a 'slip' or palpable 'clunk' as the tibia glides on the femur in an anterior cruciate deficient knee joint. An expected positive response from this test is a 'slip', 'jerk' or 'clunk' at around 10–20° of knee flexion.

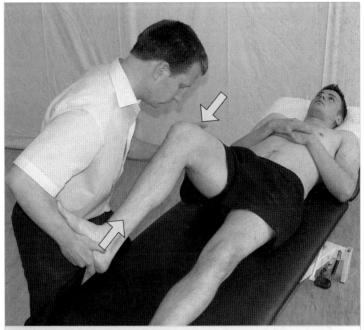

Fig 7.6   Pivot shift test. The clinician maintains a valgus force to knee joint.

PROCEDURE

Patient: The patient is positioned in long sitting or supine on a plinth. Their hip is positioned in 50–70° flexion, the knee in 45° flexion. The limb is supported by the clinician.

Clinician: The clinician's hand applies pressure to the outer surface of the leg, just below the joint line onto the head of fibula. Their other hand stabilises the foot while a valgus force is produced by applying an inward pressure through the upper hand (Fig. 7.6). Simultaneously, a medial rotation force is applied to the lower leg as the clinician slowly extends the knee (Fig. 7.7).

FINDINGS

Positive result: An obvious 'slip', 'jerk' or 'clunk' at around 10–20° of knee flexion may suggest an anterior cruciate ligament deficiency.

Negative result: There is no biomechanical abnormality on movement of the knee joint through into full extension.

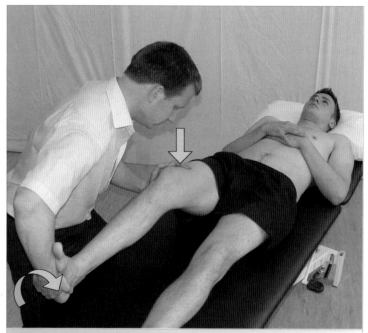

Fig 7.7 Pivot shift test. The clinician slowly extends the knee and medially rotates the knee joint assessing for a perceived 'slip', 'jerk' or 'clunk' during the movement.

Table 7.3 Sensitivity and specificity values of the pivot shift test

Author	Aim of study	Design	Sensitivity	Specificity
Benjaminse et al (2006)	To define the accuracy of clinical tests for assessing anterior cruciate ligament ruptures	Meta-analysis of 28 studies that met selection criteria	Pooled value 24%	Pooled value 98%

(table continues)

Table 7.3 (continued)

Author	Aim of study	Design	Sensitivity	Specificity
Malanga et al (2003)	To present the original descriptions of the common orthopaedic physical examination manoeuvres of the knee and a review of the literature to support the scientific validity of these tests	Meta-analysis of three studies that met the selection criteria	Range 35–98.4%	One study reported >98%
Scholten et al (2003)	Summary of the evidence on the accuracy of tests for assessing anterior cruciate ligament ruptures of the knee	Meta-analysis of 17 studies that met the selection criteria	Range 18–93%	Range 89–99%
Solomon et al (2001)	To analyse the accuracy of clinical examination findings for meniscal or ligamentous knee injuries	Meta-analysis of 23 studies that met the selection criteria	Range 27–95%	Not reported

POSTERIOR SAG SIGN

The posterior sag sign is designed to assess for a rupture of the posterior cruciate ligament. The procedure of the test involves the clinician positioning the knee into approximately 90° flexion and observing the knee from a lateral perspective. The clinician observes for a step in the knee joint line where the tibia has 'sagged' backwards due to a lack of support from the ruptured posterior cruciate ligament. An expected positive response from this test is observable 'sag' of the tibia backwards related to the femoral condyles.

PROCEDURE

Patient: The patient is positioned in long sitting on a plinth. The patient's hip is positioned in 40–50° flexion, the knee in 90° of flexion, the foot resting flat on the plinth.

Clinician: The clinician ensures that the quadriceps and hamstrings are relaxed via palpation, as slight quadriceps activity could result in a false negative result. The clinician observes the knee from the lateral aspect, follows the line from the distal end of the femoral condyles down the front of the tibia, observing for a step or sag at the knee joint line (Fig. 7.8).

FINDINGS

Positive result: A visible posterior sag of the tibia on the femur may indicate a ruptured posterior cruciate ligament.

Negative result: No evidence of a visible posterior sag suggests that the posterior cruciate ligament is intact.

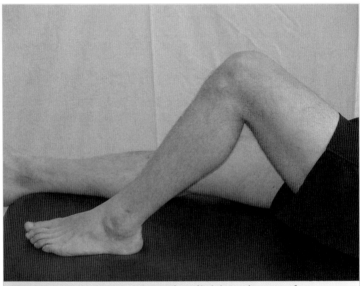

Fig 7.8   Posterior sag sign. The clinician observes for a dropping back of the tibia relative to the femur.

Table 7.4 Sensitivity and specificity values of the posterior sag test

Author	Aim of study	Design	Sensitivity	Specificity
Malanga et al (2003)	To present the original descriptions of the common orthopaedic physical examination manoeuvres of the knee and a review of the literature to support the scientific validity of these tests	Meta-analysis of one study that met the selection criteria	79%	100%

POSTERIOR DRAWER TEST

The posterior drawer test is designed to test for ligament integrity of the posterior cruciate ligament of the knee. The procedure of the test involves the clinician applying a slow, gradual anterior to posterior translation of the tibia while the knee joint is in 90° of flexion. As the posterior translation of the tibia occurs, the posterior cruciate ligament, if intact, should tighten and stop the movement. If the posterior cruciate ligament is ruptured there is no restriction to the posterior glide and this can result in an altered end feel of the movement. An expected positive response from this test is an increase in the available posterior translation of the tibia, with a corresponding alteration in the resultant end feel of the movement.

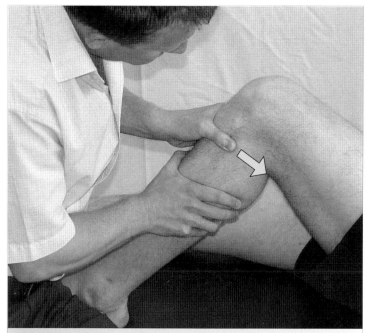

Fig 7.9 Posterior drawer test. The clinician pushes the tibia posteriorly in relation to the femur and assesses the available range and end feel of the movement.

PROCEDURE

Patient: The patient is positioned in long sitting on a plinth. Their hip is positioned in 40–50° flexion, the knee in 90° of flexion, the foot resting flat on the plinth.

Clinician: The clinician is positioned on the affected limb side, one hand stabilizing the tibia and the other hand applying an anterior posterior glide to the tibia just below the joint line (Fig. 7.9).

FINDINGS

Positive result: There is an increased glide of the tibia posteriorly, compared to the non-affected knee joint.
Negative result: The range of glide is equivocal from the affected to the non-affected knee.

Table 7.5 Sensitivity and specificity values of the posterior drawer test

Author	Aim of study	Design	Sensitivity	Specificity
Malanga et al (2003)	To present the original descriptions of the common orthopaedic physical examination manoeuvres of the knee and a review of the literature to support the scientific validity of these tests	Meta-analysis of six studies that met the selection criteria	Range 51–100%	One study reported 99%

QUADRICEPS ACTIVE TEST

The quadriceps active test is designed to test for ligament integrity of the posterior cruciate ligament of the knee. The procedure of the test involves positioning the patient in hip and knee flexion and asking the patient to contract their quadriceps. The clinician observes the knee from a lateral perspective. If the posterior cruciate ligament is ruptured the tibia will be in a 'sag' starting position and as the quadriceps contract the tibia will be drawn forwards in an anterior glide. An expected positive response from this test is an increased anterior glide of the tibia of the affected knee as the patient contracts their quadriceps.

PROCEDURE

Patient: The patient is positioned in supine on a plinth, their hip positioned in 40–50° flexion, the knee in 90° of flexion, the foot resting flat on the plinth (Fig. 7.10).

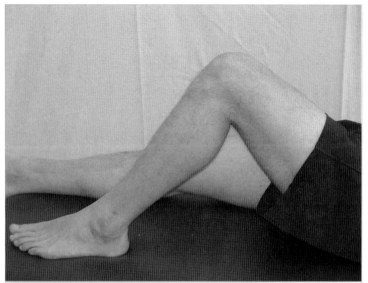

Fig 7.10   Quadriceps active test. The clinician observes the lateral aspect of the knee joint for a drawing forwards of the tibia as the patient contracts their quadriceps.

Clinician: The clinician is positioned to the side of the patient, observing the affected knee from a lateral view. The clinician asks the patient to contract their thigh muscles and watches for a possible anterior translation of the tibia.

FINDINGS

Positive result: If the tibia translates more than 2 mm it may be indicative of a posterior cruciate ligament tear and that there is excessive instability of the knee joint in a postero-anterior plane.

Negative result: If there is less than a 2 mm anterior displacement of the tibia, this may suggest a normal amount of play in the joint and therefore suggests no posterior cruciate ligament instability.

Table 7.6 Sensitivity and specificity values of the quadriceps active test

Author	Aim of study	Design	Sensitivity	Specificity
Malanga et al (2003)	To present the original descriptions of the common orthopaedic physical examination manoeuvres of the knee and a review of the literature to support the scientific validity of these tests	Meta-analysis of two studies that met the selection criteria	Range 54–98%	Range 97–100%

MEDIAL COLLATERAL LIGAMENT STRESS TEST

The medial collateral ligament stress test is designed to test the integrity of the medial collateral ligament of the knee. This test is also known as the 'valgus stress test'. The procedure involves testing the knee in two positions; 0° extension and 20–30° flexion. In both of these positions the clinician applies a valgus force, attempting to gap the medial joint line of the knee. The act of gapping the medial joint line results in a tensioning of the medial collateral ligament. The different positions provide information as to the degree of damage to the ligament and may indicate if any other structures have been damaged. An expected positive response from this test is an increase in the amount of gapping exhibited over the medial joint line and/or reproduction of the patient's symptoms.

PROCEDURE

Patient: The patient is positioned in long sitting on a plinth. This ensures that the quadriceps and hamstrings muscle groups are relaxed.

Clinician: The clinician is positioned on the side of the limb to be tested, one hand supporting the thigh and taking the weight of the upper leg. The other hand is grasping the medial aspect of the calf or ankle. This produces a length of lever mechanical advantage, enabling the clinician to impart a distraction force to the medial aspect of the knee joint. This test is performed at 0° extension (Fig. 7.11) and 20–30° flexion

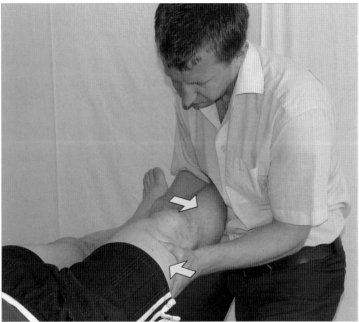

Fig 7.11   Medial collateral ligament stress test. The clinician applies a valgus force to the knee in 0° extension and assesses for laxity.

(Fig. 7.12). The clinician must then compare findings with the non-affected knee.

FINDINGS
  Positive result:
- At 20°, pain over the medial joint line with no laxity may suggest mild injury to the medial collateral ligament.
- At 20°, pain over the medial joint line and some laxity on testing may suggest a moderate injury where the ligament's integrity is compromised but it is still partially intact.
- At 20°, pain and gross instability, which is often perceived by visual gapping of the medial joint line, may suggest a complete rupture of the medial collateral ligament.
- At 0°, any instability in this position suggests that there may be a medial collateral ligament tear and cruciate ligament involvement. The knee should be stable in 0°, even with a complete rupture of the medial collateral ligament.

Negative result: No pain or laxity evident at 0° extension or 20–30° flexion, findings equivocal, as the non-affected knee.

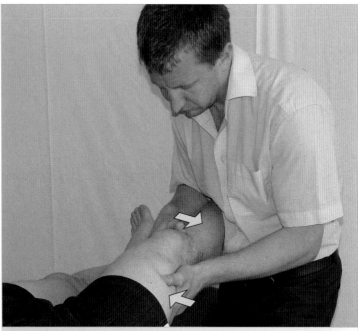

Fig 7.12 Medial collateral ligament stress test. The clinician applies a valgus force to the knee in 20° flexion and assesses for laxity.

Table 7.7 Sensitivity and specificity values of the valgus stress test

Author	Aim of study	Design	Sensitivity	Specificity
Malanga et al (2003)	To present the original descriptions of the common orthopaedic physical examination manoeuvres of the knee and a review of the literature to support the scientific validity of these tests	Meta-analysis of three studies that met the selection criteria	Range 86–96%	Not reported

LATERAL COLLATERAL LIGAMENT STRESS TEST

The lateral collateral ligament stress test is designed to test the integrity of the lateral collateral ligament of the knee. This test is also known as the 'varus stress test'. The procedure involves testing the knee in two positions: 0° extension and 20–30° flexion. In both of these positions the clinician applies a varus force, attempting to gap the lateral joint line of the knee. The act of gapping the lateral joint line results in a tensioning of the lateral collateral ligament. The different positions provide information as to the degree of damage to the ligament and may indicate if any other structures have been damaged. An expected positive response from this test is an increase in the amount of gapping exhibited over the lateral joint line and/or reproduction of the patient's symptoms.

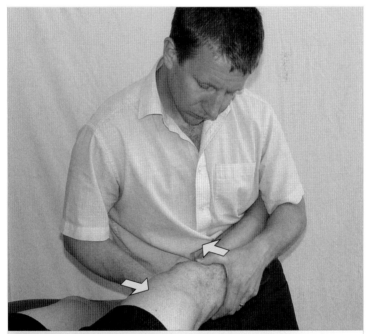

Fig 7.13 Lateral collateral ligament stress test. The clinician applies a varus force to the knee in 0° extension and assesses for laxity.

PROCEDURE

Patient: The patient is positioned in long sitting towards the edge of the plinth. Their hip is abducted so that the clinician can position themselves on the medial aspect of the leg. The leg is supported by the clinician to ensure the quadriceps and hamstring muscle groups are relaxed. This test is performed at 0° extension (Fig. 7.13) and 20–30° flexion (Fig. 7.14).

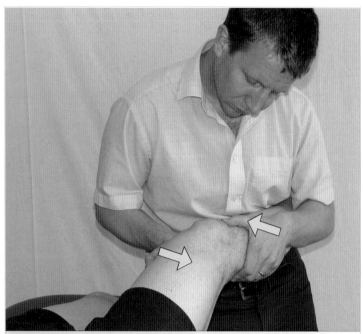

Fig 7.14 Lateral collateral ligament stress test. The clinician applies a varus force to the knee in 20° flexion and assesses for laxity.

Clinician: The clinician is positioned in standing, one hand supporting the medial and underside of the thigh above the medial joint line. The clinician's other hand grasps the outer surface of the calf towards the ankle so that a mechanical advantage of lever length can be applied in the gapping of the lateral joint line.

FINDINGS

Positive result:

- At 20°, pain over the lateral joint line with no laxity may suggest mild injury to the lateral collateral ligament.
- At 20°, pain over the lateral joint line and some laxity on testing may suggest a moderate injury where the ligament's integrity is compromised but it is still partially intact.
- At 20°, pain and gross instability, which is often perceived by visual gapping of the lateral joint line, may suggest a complete rupture of the lateral collateral ligament.
- At 0°, any instability in this position suggests that there may be a lateral collateral ligament tear and cruciate ligament involvement.

Negative result: No pain or laxity evident at 0° extension or 20–30° flexion, findings equivocal, as the non-affected knee.

Table 7.8 Sensitivity and specificity values of the varus stress test

Author	Aim of study	Design	Sensitivity	Specificity
Malanga et al (2003)	To present the original descriptions of the common orthopaedic physical examination manoeuvres of the knee and a review of the literature to support the scientific validity of these tests	Meta-analysis of one study that met the selection criteria	25%	Not reported

McMURRAY'S TEST

McMurray's test is designed to test the integrity of the menisci within the knee joint. The procedure of the test involves the clinician applying a valgus and rotational movement to the patient's knee as it is moved from flexion through to extension. The test is repeated with a varus force. The combination of the applied forces attempts to grind the medial and lateral menisci between the respective femoral and tibial condyles. If a meniscal tear is present the test may 'catch' the torn part of the meniscus. One important aspect to remember is that patellofemoral joint pathology can produce similar findings to a torn meniscus. Clarification of the mechanism of injury and other symptoms are essential in the differentiation of a meniscus tear and patellofemoral joint pathology. An expected positive response from this test is an audible 'click' or 'pop' with reported pain during the test.

PROCEDURE

Patient: The patient is positioned in supine on a plinth. The patient should be positioned close to the edge of the plinth on the side to be tested.

Clinician: The clinician is positioned in standing on the side of the knee to be tested. The clinician's hand is supporting the patient's thigh above the knee joint line. The clinician's other hand grasps the foot around the ankle, so that lateral rotation

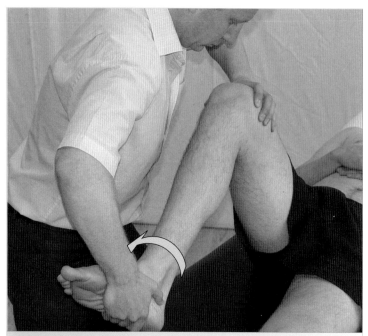

Fig 7.15 McMurray's test. The clinician fixes the knee with one hand and applies lateral rotation to the knee with the other.

(Fig. 7.15) of the tibia on the femur can be applied. The clinician then applies medial rotation (Fig. 7.16) with medial glide of the lower leg, in small sweeping movements, thus attempting to close the medial joint space and grind or catch the meniscus between the femoral and tibial condyles. The movement is repeated for the lateral compartment only with a lateral glide and lateral rotation of the tibia. These movements are performed while moving the knee from full flexion to extension. The clinician should then compare the results to the other side.

FINDINGS

Positive result: An audible 'click' or 'pop' with reported pain may suggest a tear of either the medial or the lateral meniscus.
Negative result: No audible click or pop.

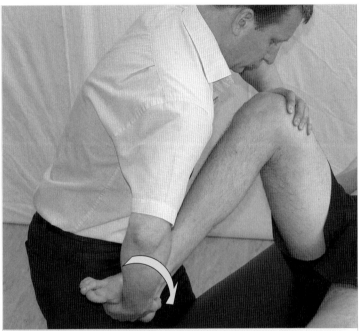

Fig 7.16   McMurray's test. The clinician then attempts to grind the meniscus between the femoral and tibial condyles by applying medial rotation in different ranges of flexion through to extension.

Table 7.9 Sensitivity and specificity values of McMurray's test

Author	Aim of study	Design	Sensitivity	Specificity
Malanga et al (2003)	To present the original descriptions of the common orthopaedic physical examination manoeuvres of the knee and a review of the literature to support the scientific validity of these tests	Meta-analysis of four studies that met the selection criteria	Range 16–58%	Range 77–98%
Scholten et al (2001)	Summary of the evidence on the accuracy of physical diagnostic tests for assessing meniscal lesions of the knee	Meta-analysis of 8 studies that met the selection criteria	Range 10–66%	Range 57–98%

(*table continues*)

Table 7.9 (continued)

Author	Aim of study	Design	Sensitivity	Specificity
Solomon et al (2001)	To analyse the accuracy of clinical examination findings for meniscal or ligamentous knee injuries	Meta-analysis of 23 studies that met the selection criteria	Range 29–63% Mean 53%	Range 29–100% Mean 59%

THESSALY TEST

The Thessaly test is designed to test the integrity of the menisci within the knee joint. The procedure of the test involves the patient standing on one leg while being supported by the clinician. The clinician instructs the patient to swivel upon a slightly flexed knee on the weight-bearing leg. This action acts to medially and laterally rotate the femur on the tibia. The combination of the applied forces attempts to grind the medial and lateral menisci between the respective femoral and tibial condyles. If a meniscal tear is present the test may 'catch' the torn part of the meniscus. An expected positive response from this test is a reproduction of a perceived 'locking' or 'catching' during the application of the test.

PROCEDURE
Patient: The patient is positioned in standing with support from the clinician.
Clinician: The clinician is positioned in front of patient, holding on to the patient's hands to provide support (Fig. 7.17). The clinician asks the patient to rotate medially and laterally (Fig. 7.18) three times while keeping the knee in slight flexion; this is then repeated while in approximately 20° knee flexion (20° flexion appears to be more effective at highlighting a possible lesion of the meniscus).

FINDINGS
Positive result: Pain over the medial or lateral joint line may indicate a possible tear of the medial or lateral meniscus respectively; the patient may also complain of a 'locking' or 'catching' sensation in the knee during the test, which may represent the catching of the meniscus between the femoral and tibial articulations.
Negative result: No reproduction of the locking or catching sensation.

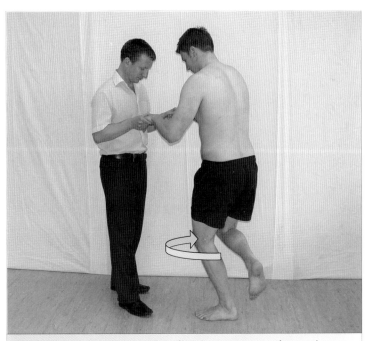

Fig 7.17   Thessaly test. The clinician supports the patient into single leg balance and slight knee flexion.

Notes

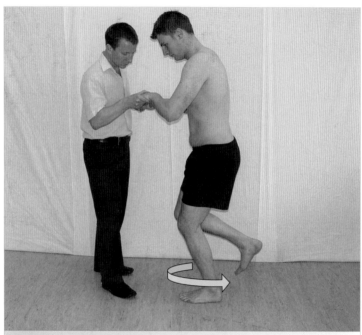

Fig 7.18 Thessaly test. The patient then medially and laterally rotates on the knee as the clinician monitors for symptom reproduction.

Table 7.10 Sensitivity and specificity values of the Thessaly test

Author	Aim of study	Design	Sensitivity	Specificity
Karachalios et al (2005)	To evaluate the diagnostic accuracy of the Thessaly test for the detection of meniscal tears	Prospective analysis of 213 subjects' Thessaly test findings with MRI findings	At 5° knee flexion 66% medial meniscus, 81% lateral meniscus At 20° knee flexion 89% medial meniscus, 92% lateral meniscus	At 5° knee flexion 96% medial meniscus, 91% lateral meniscus At 20° knee flexion 97% medial meniscus, 96% lateral meniscus

APLEY'S GRIND TEST

Apley's grind test is designed to test the integrity of the menisci within the knee joint. The procedure of the test involves the clinician applying rotation and traction or rotation and compression to the knee joint. The clinician first gaps the knee joint space by imparting traction of the tibia and then adding medial and lateral rotation. Secondly, the clinician compresses the knee joint space and applies medial and lateral rotation. If a meniscal tear is present the test may 'catch' the torn part of the meniscus during the compressive phase of the test. An expected positive response from this test is pain during the compression stage of the test.

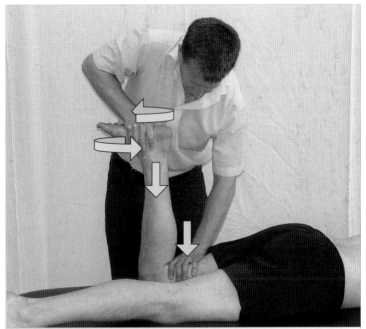

Fig 7.19 Apley's grind test. The clinician applies a vertical pull to distract the knee joint and performs medial and lateral rotation.

PROCEDURE
Patient: The patient is positioned in prone on a plinth, their knee flexed to 90°.

Clinician:

- *Stage 1*: The clinician, who is positioned in standing on the side to be tested, places their hand over the posterior aspect of the thigh as close to the posterior aspect of the knee as possible. The other hand grasps the foot around the ankle and imparts a vertical pull; this in turn will produce a distraction force to the knee. With the distraction force maintained, the clinician medially and laterally rotates the foot and thus the tibia on the femur, resulting in the tibia being medially and laterally rotated on the femur (Fig. 7.19).

- *Stage 2*: This is similar to stage 1, except the clinician applies a compression force down through the line of the tibia, resulting in a compression of the knee joint, and then continues to apply a medial and lateral rotational movement via distal tibia rotation. The clinician then assesses the opposite knee (Fig. 7.20).

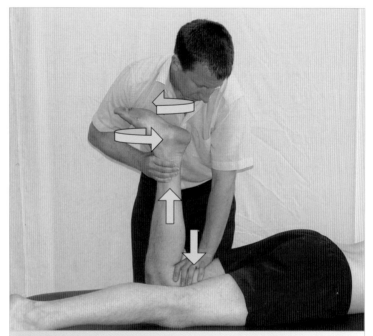

Fig 7.20 Apley's grind test. The clinician applies a compression force to the knee joint and performs medial and lateral rotation.

FINDINGS

Positive result: Pain reported during the application of stage 2, but absent during stage 1, may suggest a meniscal tear. This is due to the increased compression being more likely to catch or grind the meniscus between the femur and the tibia.

Negative result: No pain reported on the compression stage of the test.

Table 7.11 Sensitivity and specificity values of Apley's grind test

Author	Aim of study	Design	Sensitivity	Specificity
Malanga et al (2003)	To present the original descriptions of the common orthopaedic physical examination manoeuvres of the knee and a review of the literature to support the scientific validity of these tests	Meta-analysis of two studies that met the selection criteria	Range 13–16%	Range 80–90%
Scholten et al (2001)	Summary of the evidence on the accuracy of physical diagnostic tests for assessing meniscal lesions of the knee	Meta-analysis of 3 studies that met the selection criteria	Range 16–58%	Range 80–99%
Solomon et al (2001)	To analyse the accuracy of clinical examination findings for meniscal or ligamentous knee injuries	Meta-analysis of 23 studies that met the selection criteria	16%	Not recorded

JOINT LINE TENDERNESS TEST

The joint line tenderness test is designed to test for a potential meniscal tear in the knee joint. The procedure involves accurate palpation of the medial and lateral joint lines of the knee by the clinician. The clinician may palpate the knee joint line in different ranges of knee flexion, which improves accessibility to different aspects of the medial and lateral meniscus situated on their respective tibial plateau. An expected positive response from this test is the reproduction of pain over the torn meniscus site.

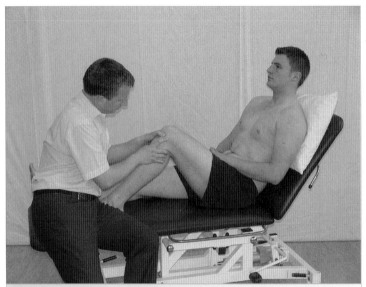

Fig 7.21 Joint line tenderness test. The clinician palpates the knee joint line and assesses for symptom reproduction.

PROCEDURE

Patient: The patient is positioned in long sitting on a plinth. Their knee is positioned in 90° flexion, their hip 40° flexion, and their foot flat on the plinth.

Clinician: The clinician is positioned on the side of the knee to be tested. The clinician stabilizes the ankle and foot to enable medial and lateral rotation as required. The finger and thumb over the top of the knee are positioned so that they can palpate the knee joint line (Fig. 7.21).

FINDINGS

Positive result: Tenderness, or occasionally a palpable mass directly on the joint line, may indicate a meniscal tear.

Negative result: No tenderness or palpable abnormality of the knee joint line.

Table 7.12 Sensitivity and specificity values of the joint line tenderness test

Author	Aim of study	Design	Sensitivity	Specificity
Malanga et al (2003)	To present the original descriptions of the common orthopaedic physical examination manoeuvres of the knee and a review of the literature to support the scientific validity of these tests	Meta-analysis of three studies that met the selection criteria	Range 55–85%	Range 29.4–67%
Scholten et al (2001)	Summary of the evidence on the accuracy of physical diagnostic tests for assessing meniscal lesions of the knee	Meta-analysis of 9 studies that met the selection criteria	Range 28–95%	Range 5–95%
Solomon et al (2001)	To analyse the accuracy of clinical examination findings for meniscal or ligamentous knee injuries	Meta-analysis of 23 studies that met the selection criteria	Range 76–85% Mean 79%	Range 11–43% Mean 15%

BOUNCE HOME TEST

The bounce home test is designed to test for a potential meniscal tear in the knee joint; it may also aid in the identification of other joint pathology, such as the presence of a loose body or a sign of swelling within the knee joint. The procedure involves the clinician applying a hyperextension force to the knee joint from a starting position of slight flexion. In a normal knee the knee joint should completely lock into extension with a firm, solid end feel. A restriction to full extension may indicate a potential obstruction within the joint. An expected positive response from this test is a restriction and a spongy or springy end feel to full knee extension.

PROCEDURE
Patient: The patient is positioned in long sitting on a plinth. Their knee is positioned in slight flexion (Fig. 7.22).

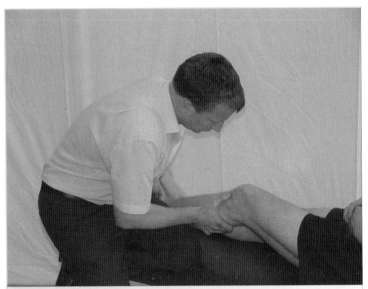

Fig 7.22 Bounce home test. The clinician supports a relaxed knee in slight flexion.

Notes

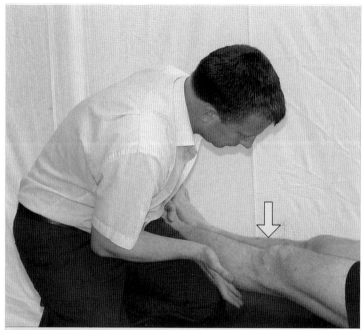

Fig 7.23 Bounce home test. The clinician releases the knee to drop into extension and assesses for any restriction to the end feel.

Clinician: The clinician is positioned in standing on the side of the knee to be tested. The clinician's hand cups the ankle. The other hand is positioned under the patient's thigh. The clinician, from this position, can drop the knee from slight flexion into full extension, assessing the quality and end feel of the movement (Fig. 7.23). For further analysis, the clinician can also apply a hyperextension force to the knee by pushing down on the quadriceps just above the knee joint.

FINDINGS

Positive result: A restriction into full extension, with a spongy or springy end feel to the movement, may suggest a meniscal tear or other intra-articular pathology.

Negative result: No restriction and a normal solid end feel to extension of the knee.

PATELLOFEMORAL GRIND TEST

The patellofemoral grind test is designed to test for pain arising from the patellofemoral joint. This test is also known as 'Clarke's sign'. The procedure of the test involves the clinician grasping the patella and applying a cephalad or caudad glide. It can be performed passively or the clinician can ask the patient to contract their quadriceps to aid in the compressive and cephalad glide. As the movement occurs the articular tissue and the articular surfaces are compressed together and thus it may initiate pain by compressing pathological structures. An expected positive response from this test is the reproduction of the patient's symptoms.

PROCEDURE 1
   Patient: The patient is positioned in long sitting on a plinth. Their knee is fully extended and the quadriceps muscles are relaxed.
   Clinician: Standing alongside the patient, the clinician grasps the apex or base of patella with the thumb and first finger, and the webspace between. A cephalad (Fig. 7.24) and caudad (Fig. 7.25)

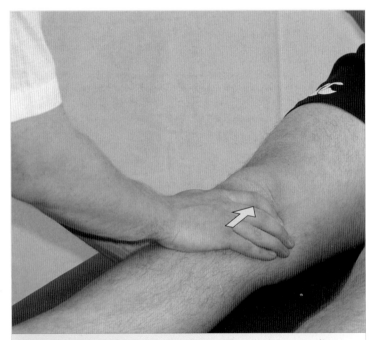

Fig 7.24 Patellofemoral grind test. The clinician applies a cephalad glide to the patella and monitors the symptoms.

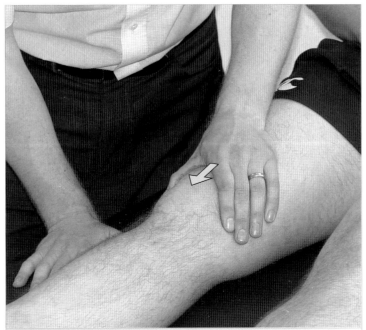

Fig 7.25   Patellofemoral grind test. The clinician applies a caudal glide to the patella and assesses for symptom reproduction.

movement is applied, respectively, to the clinician's hand position. The clinician tests the opposite knee.

PROCEDURE 2

Patient: The patient is positioned in supine or half long sitting on a plinth. Their knee flexed to 30° and the quadriceps muscles are relaxed.

Clinician: The clinician applies the caudal glide to the patella as above, and then also asks the patient to contract their quadriceps. The contraction of quadriceps results in an active pull of the patella against the femoral surface. The clinician tests the opposite knee.

FINDINGS

Positive result: Pain or reproduction of the patient's symptoms is elicited on initiation of either test procedure. Crepitus may also be heard or palpated during the test, which may be indicative of patellofemoral joint degeneration or other pathological changes taking place.

Negative result: No reproduction of symptoms.

PATELLA APPREHENSION TEST

The patella apprehension test is designed to test for instability of the patellofemoral joint. This test is also known as 'Fairbank's apprehension test'. The procedure of the test involves the clinician applying a passive medial to lateral glide of the patella in a relaxed flexed knee. As lateral dislocation or subluxation of the patella is more common, this test attempts to replicate the direction of dislocation or subluxation and thus may produce a feeling of anxiety or apprehension in the patient. It should be remembered that this test may also produce symptoms in a patient who presents with patellofemoral joint pain from another potential pathological source. An expected positive response from this test is a reported feeling of apprehension from the patient.

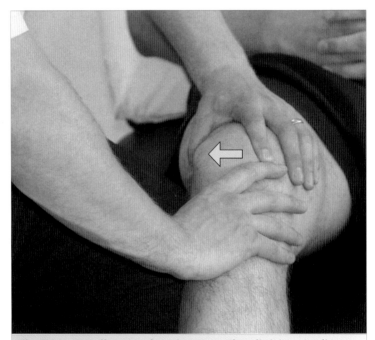

Fig 7.26 Patella apprehension test. The clinician applies a lateral glide to the patella and monitors for symptoms of apprehension from the patient.

PROCEDURE

Patient: The patient is positioned in long sitting on a plinth. Their hip is positioned in 30° flexion, the knee in 30° of flexion.
Clinician: The clinician is positioned alongside the patient. Their knee is positioned on the plinth, supporting the patient's knee. The fingers or thumbs of both hands are placed on the medial edge of the patella, applying a medial to lateral glide of the patella (Fig. 7.26). The clinician monitors the patient's reaction. The clinician assesses both knees to compare findings.

FINDINGS

Positive result: A reported feeling of apprehension by the patient may suggest instability of the patellofemoral joint. The test may also reproduce the patient's pain or symptoms.
Negative result: No apprehension or reproduction of symptoms.

Table 7.13 Sensitivity and specificity values of the patella apprehension test

Author	Aim of study	Design	Sensitivity	Specificity
Malanga et al (2003)	To present the original descriptions of the common orthopaedic physical examination manoeuvres of the knee and a review of the literature to support the scientific validity of these tests	Meta-analysis of one study that met the selection criteria	39%	Not reported

REFERENCES

Benjaminse A, Gokeler A, van der Schans C 2006 Clinical diagnosis of an anterior cruciate ligament rupture: a meta-analysis. Journal of Orthopaedic and Sports Physical Therapy 36(5): 267–288

Karachalios T, Hantes M, Zibis A et al 2005 Diagnostic accuracy of a new clinical test (the Thessaly test) for early detection of meniscal tears. Journal of Bone and Joint Surgery 87(5): 955–962

Malanga G, Andrus S, Nadler S et al 2003 Physical examination of the knee: a review of the original test description and scientific validity of common orthopaedic tests. Archives of Physical Medicine and Rehabilitation 84(4): 592–603

Scholten R, Deville W, Opstelten W et al 2001 The accuracy of physical diagnostic tests for assessing meniscal lesions of the knee: a meta-analysis. Journal of Family Practice 50(11): 938–944

Scholten R, Opstelten W, van der Plas C et al 2003 Accuracy of physical diagnostic tests for assessing ruptures of the anterior cruciate ligament: a meta-analysis. Journal of Family Practice 52(9): 689–694

Solomon D, Simel D, Bates D et al 2001 Does this patient have a torn meniscus or ligament of the knee? Journal of the American Medical Association 286(13): 1610–1620

BIBLIOGRAPHY AND FURTHER READING

Magee D 2008 Orthopedic physical assessment, 5th edn. Saunders Elsevier, St Louis, MO

Norris C 2005 Sports injuries diagnosis and management, 3rd edn. Butterworth-Heinemann, Edinburgh

The ankle

ANTERIOR DRAWER TEST

The anterior drawer test is designed to test for instability of the ankle joint by assessing the integrity of the surrounding ligaments. The procedure of the test involves applying a posterior to anterior movement of the talus on the tibia and fibula. The anterior translation of the talus tensions the surrounding ligaments which restricts the amount of glide available. If the ligament integrity has been compromised there may be an increased range of anterior draw and possible alterations in the end feel of the movement. A slight alteration of the ankle position during testing may help to differentiate which ligament has been affected. An expected positive response from this test is the identification of increased anterior translation of the talus within the talo-crural joint, together with a possible alteration of the end feel of the movement. The test may also reproduce the patient's symptoms.

PROCEDURE

Patient: The patient is positioned in long sitting on a plinth. Their hip is positioned at 40° flexion, their knee in 90° of flexion, and their foot flat on the plinth, resulting in approximately 10–20° plantarflexion of the ankle.

Clinician: The clinician stands at the base of the plinth, one hand supporting the dorsum of the foot and the other positioned just above the superior joint line of the ankle. The clinician then

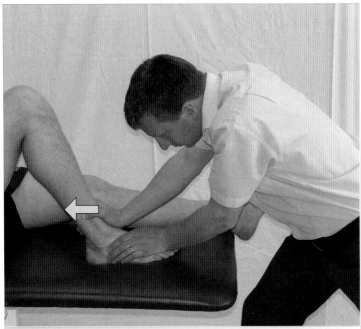

Fig 8.1 Anterior drawer test. The clinician applies a posteriorly directed force to the tibia while fixing the talus. This results in a relative anterior translation of the talus within the ankle joint.

applies an anterior to posterior force through the tibia and fibula to produce a relative postero-anterior glide of the talus on the tibia and fibula (Fig. 8.1). The clinician compares the results to the non-affected side.

FINDINGS

Positive result: An increased anterior glide of the talus in the joint complex may suggest a level of instability in the joint, due to a lack of ligament integrity. A soft end feel to the movement may also indicate instability of the ankle joint.

Negative result: No difference in the amount of anterior glide of the talus compared to the non-affected side.

TALAR TILT TEST

The talar tilt test is designed to test for instability of the ankle joint by assessing the available angle of movement between the head of the talus and the distal articular surface of the tibia. The angle produced by the head of the talus and the distal articular surface of the tibia is normally reported to be between 5° and 23°. However, after ligament disruption the affected ankle may have a much larger talar tilt angle on the affected side. This increase in talar tilt angle may occur due to the lack of restraint, normally provided by the lateral ligament complex of the ankle. An expected positive response from the test is an increase of the talar tilt angle by 10° or more, compared to the non-affected side. The test may also reproduce the patient's symptoms.

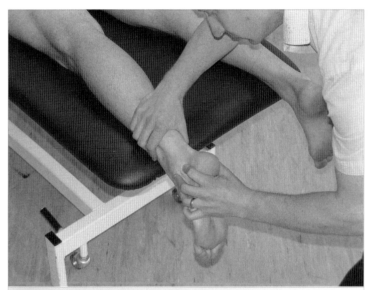

Fig 8.2   Talar tilt test. The clinician fixes the tibia and fibula with one hand while gripping the talus with the other.

PROCEDURE

Patient: The patient is positioned in prone on a plinth with their legs hanging over the end of the plinth.

Clinician: The clinician is positioned at the foot of the plinth at the foot of the plinth. One hand stabilizes the medial aspect of the patient's leg, grasping the tibial shaft, allowing enough space for inversion of the ankle (Fig. 8.2). Their other hand is placed under the foot, grasping the calcaneus with the palm and with the

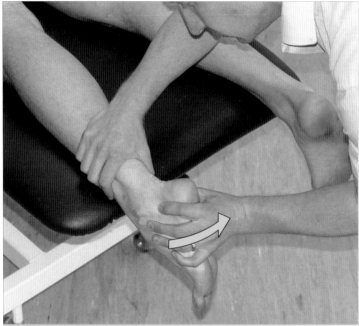

Fig 8.3 Talar tilt test. The clinician then tilts the talus medially and assesses the range of movement available.

fingers encapsulating the calcaneus and talus. The clinician then inverts the talus, keeping the tibia and fibula fixed (Fig. 8.3). This provides good stabilization of the calcaneus and talus, preventing a false movement, and also allows differentiation between the talar and subtalar joint, resulting in a more isolated movement of the talus in the crural space.

FINDINGS

Positive result: A positive result is identified when the affected ankle moves 10° or more than the non-affected ankle. Symptom reproduction information from the patient may also provide some feedback as to the position of their pain or discomfort; however, primarily, an increase in the talar tilt angle may be indicative of ligament damage.

Negative result: No difference in the talar tilt angle from the affected ankle to the non-affected ankle. Similarly, there may be no symptom reproduction.

SYNDESMOSIS SQUEEZE TEST

The syndesmosis squeeze test is designed to test for a syndesmosis injury. A syndesmosis injury is often referred to as a high sprain of the ankle where the injury and the tissues damaged are different to those of a typical lateral ligament sprain. As the ankle inverts, the force is applied through the movement of the talus which acts to gap the tibia and fibula. This can lead to disruption of the ligaments and the interosseous structures between the two bones. The procedure of the test involves the clinician gently squeezing the tibia and the fibula together. This force acts directly on the tibia and fibula and their connecting soft tissues more than the ankle joint complex. An expected positive response from this test is the reproduction of the patient's pain or symptoms.

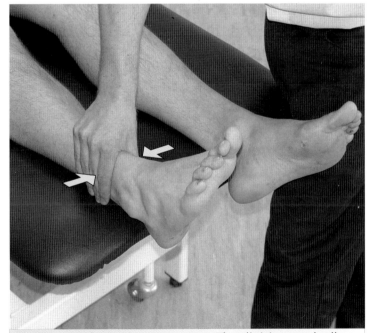

Fig 8.4 Syndesmosis squeeze test. The clinician gradually squeezes the tibia and fibula together just above the ankle joint line and assesses for symptom reproduction.

PROCEDURE

Patient: The patient is positioned in long sitting on a plinth.

Clinician: The clinician is positioned at the foot of the plinth adjacent to the ankle to be tested. Their hand gently grasps the patient's tibia and fibula, proximal to the ankle joint line. The other hand supports the limb if necessary. The clinician gently squeezes the tibia and fibula, monitors for symptom reproduction, and compares the findings to the opposite side (Fig. 8.4).

FINDINGS

Positive result: Pain or reproduction of the patient's pain over the syndesmotic ligaments in the ankle may suggest a syndesmosis injury.

Negative result: No pain initiated on testing.

THOMPSON TEST

The Thompson test is designed to test the integrity of the Achilles tendon. This test is also known as 'Simmons test' and the 'calf squeeze test'. The procedure of the test involves the clinician applying a gentle squeeze to the calf muscle belly. This action creates a pull on the Achilles tendon and on to its attachment into the calcaneus, thus resulting in an observable plantarflexion of the ankle. If the tendon has been ruptured the calf squeeze does not initiate a corresponding plantarflexion of the ankle. The clinician should note that there could be a partial tear of the tendon, which may produce a negative result but should still be considered a serious pathology. Furthermore, in the event of a complete tear the test may still potentially produce a negative finding. An expected positive response from the test is the failure for the ankle to move into plantarflexion as the calf is squeezed.

PROCEDURE

Patient: The patient is positioned in prone with both feet overhanging the end of the plinth. There should be sufficient space to allow for some degree of plantarflexion without restriction of movement from the plinth. The clinician should ensure that the patient remains relaxed.

Clinician: The clinician is positioned standing alongside the affected ankle of the patient, towards the foot of the plinth.

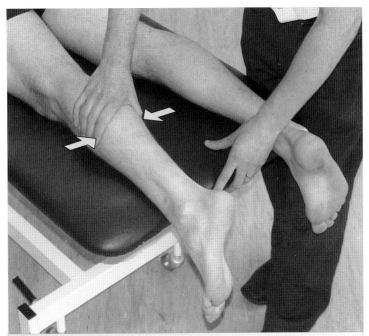

Fig 8.5 Thompson test. The clinician squeezes the muscle bulk of the calf.

The clinician gently places their hand over the bulk of the calf muscle, and applies a gradual squeeze to the muscle bulk (Fig. 8.5). Clear observation of the foot is essential. As the calf is squeezed, the foot moves into plantarflexion if the tendon is intact (Fig. 8.6). If unsure, the other hand can lightly touch the sole of the foot to assess for any movement, but realistically if the tendon is intact the movement into plantarflexion is clearly apparent. The clinician compares the affected side to the opposite side.

FINDINGS

Positive result: There will be no movement of the foot into plantarflexion when the calf muscle bulk is squeezed, suggesting a complete tear or rupture of the Achilles tendon.

Negative result: The foot moves equally into plantarflexion as the non-affected side, suggesting that there is no rupture of the tendon.

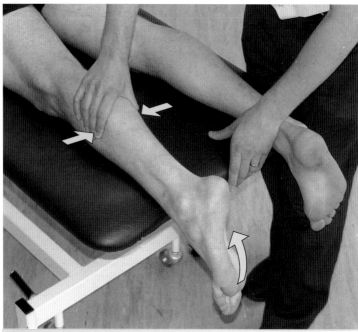

Fig 8.6 Thompson test. The clinician assesses for associated plantarflexion of the ankle to establish Achilles tendon integrity.

Table 8.1 Sensitivity and specificity values of the Thompson test

Author	Aim of study	Design	Sensitivity	Specificity
Maffulli (1998)	To determine the sensitivity and specificity of several clinical diagnostic tests for unilateral subcutaneous Achilles tendon rupture	Correlation of 174 subjects' calf squeeze test findings with open repair of the Achilles tendon	96%	93%

REFERENCES

Maffulli N 1998 The clinical diagnosis of subcutaneous tear of the Achilles tendon: a prospective study in 174 patients. American Journal of Sports Medicine 26(2): 266–270

BIBLIOGRAPHY AND FURTHER READING

Lynch S 2002 Assessment of the injured ankle in the athlete. Journal of Athletic Training 37(4): 406–412

Magee D 2008 Orthopedic physical assessment, 5th edn. Saunders Elsevier, St Louis, MO

Norris C 2005 Sports injuries diagnosis and management, 3rd edn. Butterworth-Heinemann, Edinburgh

van Dijk C 2002 Management of the sprained ankle. British Journal of Sports Medicine 36(2): 83–84

Nerve integrity

DEEP TENDON REFLEXES

The deep tendon reflexes are designed to test the integrity of a reflex arc. The procedure of the test involves the clinician tapping a tendon of a specific muscle with a reflex hammer. The test initiates a reflex arc, which is a connection of the afferent nerve from the muscle to the spinal cord and back to the muscle via a separate nerve fibre. A stimulated reflex arc results in a characteristic reflex jerk movement when the tendon of a corresponding muscle is tapped with a reflex hammer. Normally the characteristic reflex jerk occurs on testing and the response is seen as equal when comparing the left side to the right side. An expected positive response from this test is an absent or altered reflex on the affected side or bilaterally.

FINDINGS

Positive result: An absent reflex on the affected side and a normal jerk on the unaffected side may suggest that conduction along the peripheral nerve is totally compromised. If the reflex is present on the affected side but is less reactive than the unaffected side, this may suggest that conduction has been partially compromised. The term often used for a less reactive reflex is 'hypo-reflexia'. If the reflex is present but is more reactive than normal, this may suggest a raised state of anxiety or an upper motor neurone lesion. The term often used for a more reactive reflex is 'hyper-reflexia' or 'brisk'.

BICEPS C5/6 DEEP TENDON REFLEX

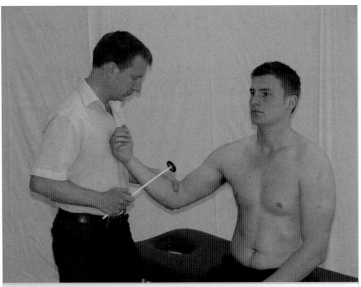

Fig 9.1 Testing the biceps deep tendon reflex.

PROCEDURE

Patient: The patient is positioned in sitting, shoulders neutral, elbow flexed to 90°.

Clinician: The clinician is positioned standing alongside the patient on the side to be tested. The clinician supports the upper limb at the elbow, maintaining the flexed elbow position. Support from the clinician is essential as the patient's muscles should be fully relaxed before testing. The clinician palpates the biceps tendon in the area of the cubital fossa and pushes their thumb on to the tendon. The clinician gently strikes their thumb once with the reflex hammer. The clinician notes the reaction and may repeat the test if required and proceeds to test the opposite side (Fig. 9.1).

TRICEPS C6 DEEP TENDON REFLEX

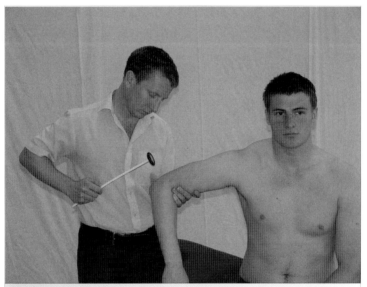

Fig 9.2   Testing the triceps deep tendon reflex.

PROCEDURE

Patient: The patient is positioned in sitting, shoulder in 90° abduction, full internal rotation, arm relaxed and supported by the clinician.

Clinician: The clinician is positioned standing alongside the patient on the side to be tested. The clinician supports the patient under the upper arm, allowing the elbow to hang in 90° flexion. The clinician palpates the triceps tendon between the end of the muscle belly and its insertion into the olecranon of the ulna. The clinician gently strikes the tendon once with the reflex hammer. The clinician notes the reaction or repeats the test if required and proceeds to test the opposite side (Fig. 9.2).

BRACHIORADIALIS C6/7 DEEP TENDON REFLEX

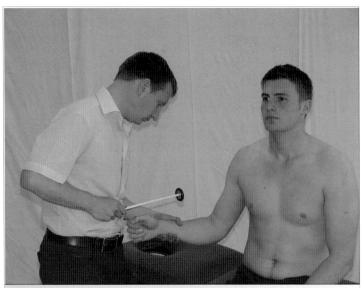

Fig 9.3 Testing the brachioradialis deep tendon reflex.

PROCEDURE

Patient: The patient is positioned in sitting, elbow flexed to 90°, forearm in the mid-position and supported by the clinician.

Clinician: The clinician is positioned standing alongside the patient on the side to be tested. The clinician supports the patient's forearm and palpates the brachioradialis tendon as it blends from the muscle belly into the tendon. The thumb rests over the tendon to provide suitable contact for the transmission of the force of the hammer. The clinician gently strikes their thumb once with the reflex hammer. The clinician notes the reaction or repeats the test if required and proceeds to test the opposite side (Fig. 9.3).

PATELLA TENDON L3/4 DEEP TENDON REFLEX

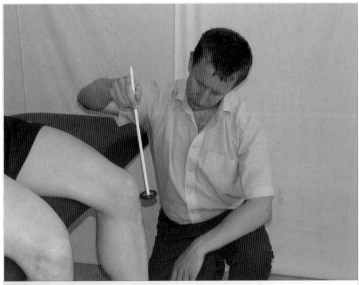

Fig 9.4   Testing the patella deep tendon reflex.

PROCEDURE

Patient: The patient is positioned in sitting on a plinth, with their feet off the floor.

Clinician: The clinician is positioned in standing alongside the patient on the side to be tested. The clinician palpates the patella tendon and strikes the tendon once with the patella hammer, making sure the hammer is perpendicular to the tendon to ensure adequate transmission of force through the tendon. The clinician notes the reaction or repeats the test if required and proceeds to test the opposite side (Fig. 9.4).

ACHILLES TENDON L5 S1 DEEP TENDON REFLEX

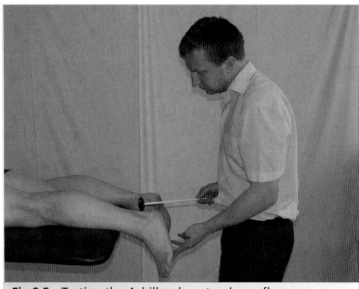

Fig 9.5 Testing the Achilles deep tendon reflex.

PROCEDURE

Patient: The patient is positioned in prone, their feet hanging over the end of the plinth.

Clinician: The clinician is positioned standing alongside the patient on the side to be tested. The clinician palpates the tendon and strikes the tendon once with the patella hammer, making sure the hammer is perpendicular to the tendon to ensure adequate transmission of force through the tendon. The clinician notes the reaction or repeats the test if required and proceeds to test the opposite side (Fig. 9.5).

MYOTOME TESTING

Myotome testing is designed to test the integrity of the nerve supply to a group of muscles. The procedure of the test consists of the clinician performing an isometric muscle strength test for a specific muscle group. The muscle group corresponds to the nerve root value of their supply as can be identified in Table 9.1 for cervical nerve roots and Table 9.2 for lumbar nerve roots. A muscle group's isometric muscle strength relates directly to the nerve root innervation, and thus may aid in the identification of the potential root level of a nerve lesion. An expected positive result is a loss or weakness in isometric muscle strength, either unilaterally or bilaterally. A guide to the testing procedure for cervical and lumbar myotomes can be identified in the subsequent pages.

Table 9.1 Cervical myotomes

Nerve root	Muscle group
C1	Neck flexors
C2	Neck extensors
C3	Neck side flexors
C4	Shoulder girdle elevators
C5	Shoulder abductors
C6	Elbow flexors
C7	Elbow extensors
C8	Thumb extensors
T1	Finger abductors

Table 9.2 Lumbar myotomes

Nerve root	Muscle group
L2	Hip flexors
L3	Knee extensors
L4	Ankle dorsiflexors and invertors
L5	Toe extensors
S1	Foot evertors
S2	Ankle plantarflexors
S1 and S2	Knee flexors

FINDINGS

Positive result: A unilateral absence of an isometric muscle contraction for a specific muscle group may suggest a lesion, or a complete failure to conduct, of the peripheral nerve supplying that muscle group. A unilateral weakness of an isometric muscle contraction for a specific muscle group may suggest the partial failure to conduct of a peripheral nerve supplying that muscle group. Bilateral absence or weakness of a myotome may suggest a pathology affecting the nervous system centrally and may require further examination as it may suggest more serious pathology.

Negative result: Demonstration of normal muscle strength bilaterally.

CERVICAL MYOTOMES

NERVE ROOT C1 MYOTOME: NECK FLEXORS

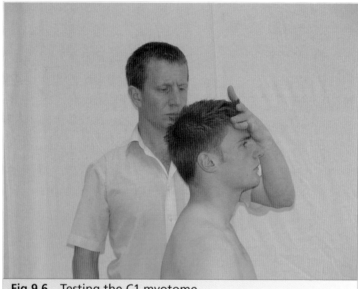

Fig 9.6 Testing the C1 myotome.

PROCEDURE

Patient: The patient is positioned in sitting with their cervical spine in neutral.

Clinician: Standing to the side of the patient, the clinician applies their hand to the patient's forehead and asks the patient to slowly build up resistance against the clinician's hand. This prevents a sudden jolt or jerking movement for the patient and thus reduces the chance of irritating the patient's symptoms (Fig. 9.6).

NERVE ROOT C2 MYOTOME: NECK EXTENSORS

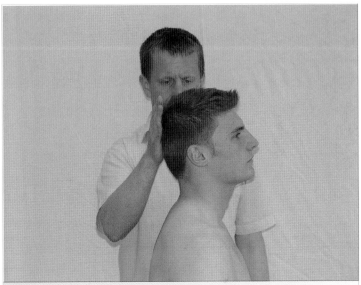

Fig 9.7 Testing the C2 myotome.

PROCEDURE

Patient: The patient is positioned in sitting with their cervical spine in neutral.

Clinician: Standing to the side of the patient, the clinician applies their hand to the patient's occipital area and asks the patient to slowly build up resistance against the clinician's hand. This prevents a sudden jolt or jerking movement for the patient and thus reduces the chance of irritating the patient's symptoms (Fig. 9.7).

NERVE ROOT C3 MYOTOME: NECK SIDE FLEXORS

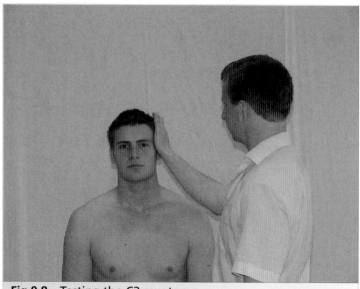

Fig 9.8   Testing the C3 myotome.

PROCEDURE

Patient: The patient is positioned in sitting with their cervical spine in neutral.

Clinician: Standing in front of the patient, the clinician applies their hand to the side of the patient's head and asks the patient to slowly build up pressure on to the clinician's hand. This prevents a sudden jolt or jerking movement for the patient and thus reduces the chance of irritating the patient's symptoms. The test is then repeated on the contralateral side (Fig. 9.8).

NERVE ROOT C4 MYOTOME: SHOULDER GIRDLE ELEVATORS

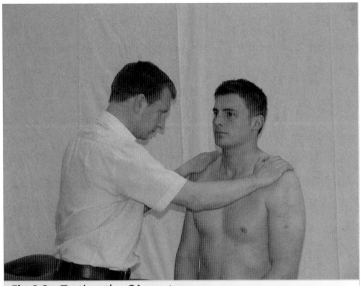

Fig 9.9   Testing the C4 myotome.

PROCEDURE

Patient: The patient is positioned in sitting with their cervical spine in neutral and their shoulders elevated half way.

Clinician: Standing in front of the patient, to test both sides simultaneously, the clinician places both hands on to the patient's shoulders and asks the patient to try and stop the clinician pushing the shoulders down. The clinician continues to apply a slow, gradual pressure to the patient's shoulders until the desired resistance is achieved (Fig. 9.9).

NERVE ROOT C5 MYOTOME: SHOULDER ABDUCTORS

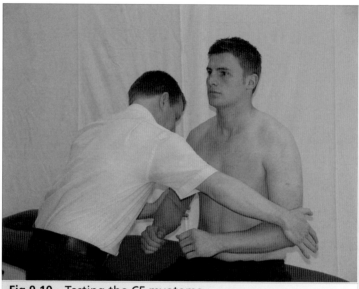

Fig 9.10 Testing the C5 myotome.

PROCEDURE

Patient: The patient is positioned in sitting with their cervical spine in neutral, their shoulders in neutral or slight flexion and elbows flexed to 90°.

Clinician: Standing in front of the patient, the clinician positions their hands on the outside of the patient's elbows and asks the patient to try and push out slowly against the clinician's hands. The clinician applies a slow, gradual pressure to the outside of the patient's arms until the desired resistance is achieved (Fig. 9.10).

NERVE ROOT C6 MYOTOME: ELBOW FLEXORS

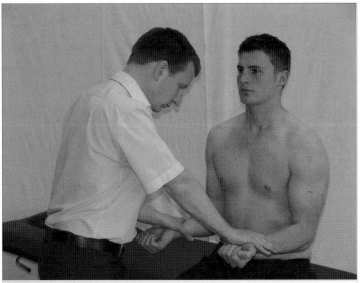

Fig 9.11   Testing the C6 myotome.

PROCEDURE

Patient: The patient is positioned in sitting with their cervical spine in neutral. Their elbows are flexed to 90° and their forearms are fully supinated.

Clinician: Standing in front of the patient, the clinician positions their hands proximal to the patient's wrists and asks the patient to try and slowly push up against the downwards resistance. The clinician applies a slow, gradual pressure to the patient's arms against the patient's elbow flexion movement until the desired resistance is achieved (Fig. 9.11).

NERVE ROOT C7 MYOTOME: ELBOW EXTENSORS

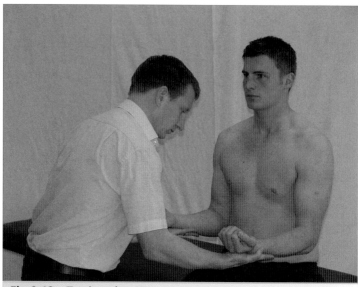

Fig 9.12 Testing the C7 myotome.

PROCEDURE

Patient: The patient is positioned in sitting with their cervical spine in neutral. Their elbows are flexed to 90° and their forearms are fully supinated.

Clinician: Standing in front of the patient, the clinician positions their hands under the patient's forearms proximal to the patient's wrists and asks the patient to try and slowly push downwards against the upwards resistance. The clinician applies a slow, gradual pressure against the patient's elbow extension until the desired resistance is achieved (Fig. 9.12).

NERVE ROOT C8 MYOTOME: THUMB EXTENSORS

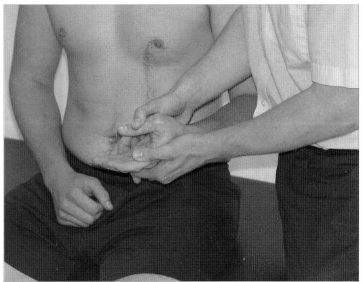

Fig 9.13   Testing the C8 myotome.

PROCEDURE

Patient: The patient is positioned in sitting. Their elbows are flexed to 90° and their forearms are fully supinated. Their thumbs are in opposition.

Clinician: Standing in front of the patient, the clinician grasps the patient's hands with the clinician's thumbs holding the patient's thumbs against their palm. The clinician asks the patient to try and push their thumbs out from their palm, thus resisting thumb extension (Fig. 9.13).

NERVE ROOT T1 MYOTOME: FINGER ABDUCTORS

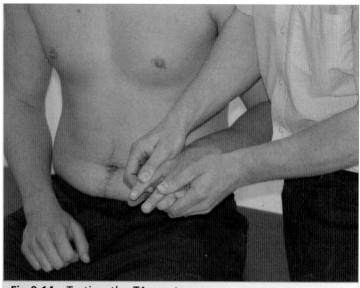

Fig 9.14   Testing the T1 myotome.

PROCEDURE

Patient: The patient is positioned in sitting. Their elbows are flexed to 90°, with their forearms pronated and their metacarpal-phalangeal joints in extension and abduction.

Clinician: Standing in front of the patient, the clinician asks the patient to try and keep their fingers spread out wide. The clinician tries to push individual fingers together with their own fingers, testing the index and middle finger first, the middle and ring finger second, and the ring and little finger last. The clinician then tests the opposite hand (Fig. 9.14).

LUMBAR MYOTOMES

NERVE ROOT L2 MYOTOME: HIP FLEXORS

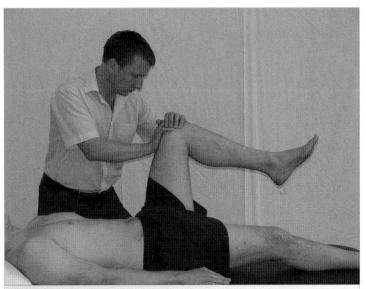

Fig 9.15   Testing the L2 myotome.

PROCEDURE

Patient: The patient is positioned in supine on a plinth, their hip in 90° flexion and knee in 90° flexion.

Clinician: Standing on the side of the patient to be tested, the clinician places both hands against the anterior aspect of the distal aspect of the thigh and asks the patient to try and push against their resistance by slowly increasing the pressure against the applied resistance. The clinician notes the results and tests the opposite side and notes any differences between the two sides (Fig. 9.15).

NERVE ROOT L3 MYOTOME: KNEE EXTENSORS

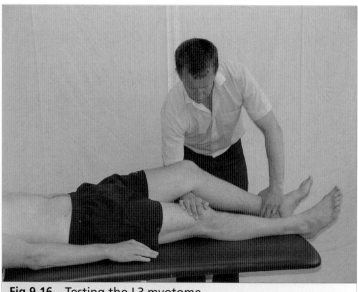

Fig 9.16 Testing the L3 myotome.

PROCEDURE

Patient: The patient is positioned in supine on a plinth, their knee in approximately 40° flexion and their foot resting on the plinth.

Clinician: Standing on the side of the patient to be tested, the clinician supports the patient's leg under the thigh and grasps around the patient's ankle with the opposite hand. The clinician asks the patient to try and extend the knee against the slow, gradual build-up of resistance applied by the clinician. The clinician notes the results and tests the opposite side and notes any differences between the two sides (Fig. 9.16).

NERVE ROOT L4 MYOTOME: ANKLE DORSIFLEXORS AND FOOT INVERTORS

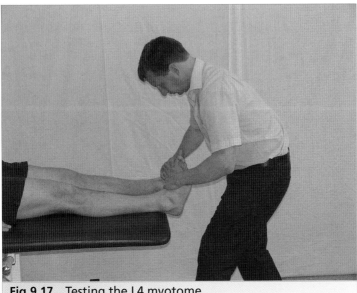

Fig 9.17 Testing the L4 myotome.

PROCEDURE

Patient: The patient is positioned in supine on a plinth.

Clinician: The clinician is standing at the foot of the plinth, applying pressure to the dorsal surface of both feet simultaneously. The clinician asks the patient to try and lift their toes up towards their head and to try and turn their foot inwards so that the soles of their feet are facing each other. The clinician resists this action and notes any differences between the left and right foot, and notes the patient's ability to perform the test (Fig. 9.17).

NERVE ROOT L5 MYOTOME: TOE EXTENSORS

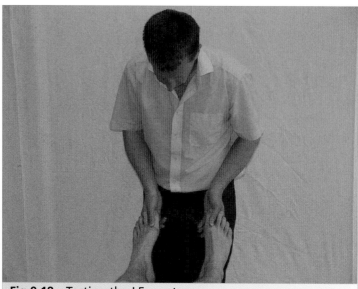

Fig 9.18 Testing the L5 myotome.

PROCEDURE

Patient: The patient is positioned in supine on a plinth.

Clinician: The clinician is standing at the foot of the plinth. The clinician places their thumbs on to the dorsal aspect of the patient's great toes and asks the patient to try and lift their toes up against the applied resistance. The clinician notes the results and notes any differences between the left and right toe extensors (Fig. 9.18).

NERVE ROOT S1 MYOTOME: FOOT EVERTORS

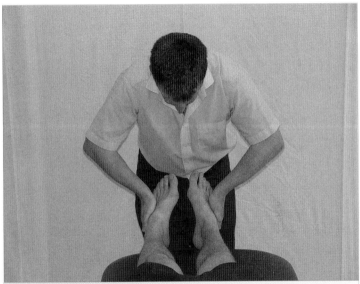

Fig 9.19 Testing the S1 myotome.

PROCEDURE

Patient: The patient is positioned in supine on a plinth.

Clinician: Standing at the foot of the plinth, applying pressure to the lateral aspect of both feet simultaneously, the clinician asks the patient to try and turn their feet outwards so that the soles of their feet are facing away from each other. The clinician resists this action and notes any differences between the left and right foot, and notes the patient's ability to perform the test (Fig. 9.19).

NERVE ROOT S1 MYOTOME: ANKLE PLANTARFLEXORS

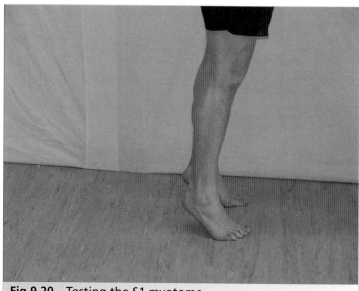

Fig 9.20 Testing the S1 myotome.

PROCEDURE

Patient: The patient is positioned in standing.

Clinician: Standing in front of the patient, holding on to the patient's hands to provide support, the clinician asks the patient to first try and stand on tip toe on both feet and hold the position. Secondly, if this has failed to identify any weakness, the clinician can test further by asking the patient to stand on tip toe on each leg independently. The patient's own body weight provides enough resistance to test for isometric muscle strength. The clinician notes the results and proceeds to test the other leg (Fig. 9.20).

NERVE ROOT S1 AND S2 MYOTOME: KNEE FLEXORS

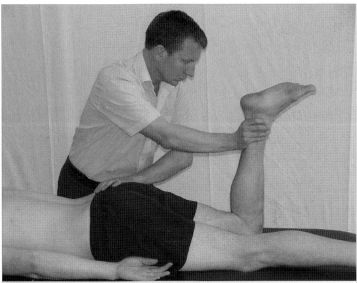

Fig 9.21   Testing the S1 and S2 myotome.

PROCEDURE

Patient: The patient is positioned in prone on a plinth. The knee to be tested is positioned in 90° flexion.

Clinician: Standing on the side to be tested, near the patient's head but facing down the plinth, the clinician grasps the posterior aspect of the patient's ankle and asks the patient to try and pull their heel up towards their buttock. Slowly the clinician gradually applies resistance to the patient's knee flexion. The clinician notes the results and proceeds to test the contralateral side (Fig. 9.21).

DERMATOME TESTING

Dermatome testing is designed to test the integrity of the nerve supply to a dermatomal area of skin. The procedure of the test involves assessing the patient's ability to perceive the sensation of light touch. The area of skin tested corresponds to the nerve root values of that area's dermatomal supply, as can be identified in Figure 9.22. A dermatomal area's ability to perceive light touch sensation relates directly to the nerve root innervation, and thus dermatomal testing may aid in the identification of the potential root level of a nerve lesion. An expected positive result is absent or diminished light touch sensation of a specific dermatomal area.

PROCEDURE

Patient: The patient is positioned in supine or sitting and should be suitably undressed to expose the dermatomal areas of skin to be tested.

Clinician: Standing alongside or in front of the patient, the clinician demonstrates the test procedure to the patient on a non-affected area first. The clinician instructs the patient to close their eyes and to say the word 'yes' when they feel the cotton wool touch their skin. The clinician identifies the dermatomes to be tested, reminds the patient of the instructions and proceeds to *lightly* dab the cotton wool on a dermatomal area, noting the patient's responses; the clinician then compares the other side. The clinician then proceeds to check light touch sensation throughout the remaining dermatomes in the same manner (Fig. 9.23).

FINDINGS

Positive result: A unilateral absence of light touch sensation of a single dermatome may suggest a lesion, or a complete failure to conduct, of a peripheral nerve supplying that dermatomal region. A unilateral lessening of light touch sensation of a single dermatomal area may suggest a partial failure of a peripheral nerve supplying that dermatomal region. Bilateral absence or lessening of light touch sensation of a dermatomal area may suggest a pathology affecting the nervous system centrally and may require further examination as this may suggest more serious pathology.

Negative result: Normal light touch sensation throughout all dermatomal areas.

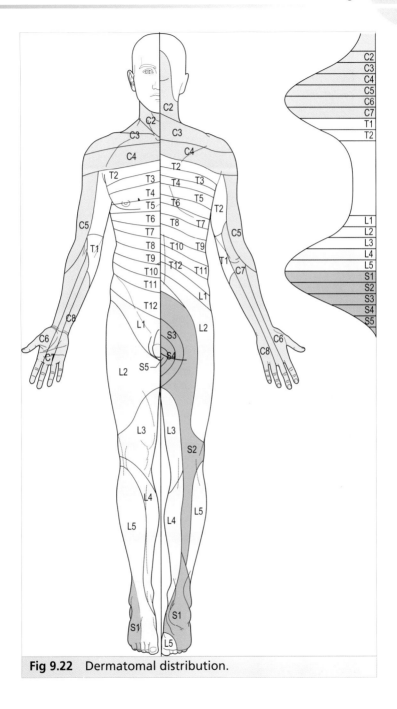

Fig 9.22   Dermatomal distribution.

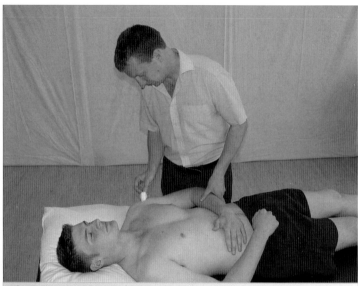

Fig 9.23 Testing a dermatome.

BIBLIOGRAPHY AND FURTHER READING

Butler D 2000 The sensitive nervous system. Noigroup Publications, Adelaide, Australia

Magee D 2008 Orthopedic physical assessment, 5th edn. Saunders Elsevier, St Louis, MO

Petty N 2006 Neuromusculoskeletal examination and assessment, 3rd edn. Elsevier, Edinburgh

Neurodynamics

NEURODYNAMIC TESTING

Neurodynamic testing is designed to test the mobility or sensitivity of the nervous system. The clinical tests are based around the concept that the peripheral and central nervous system is a mobile system. As a subject moves the neural tissue may glide between its surrounding structures. As a nerve winds around or passes through surrounding structures it may come up against points of resistance; these are often described as 'interfaces'. By application of a series of movements to test the mobility of a nerve the clinician may be able to identify a restriction in the nerve's mobility and possibly identify which interface is causing the restriction. Further development of the concept suggests that there may not necessarily be an active restriction to neural glide; a nerve that has been sensitized by trauma or pathology may also exhibit a restriction in its available glide. The base tests are described in the following chapter; however, further application and interpretation of the tests requires more familiarity with the concepts in neurodynamic testing. The reader is referred to Butler (2000) and Shacklock (2005) for a more in-depth explanation of the concept and the use of neurodynamic testing in practice.

STRAIGHT LEG RAISE

The straight leg raise is designed to test the neurodynamics or the sensitivity of the sciatic nerve. The procedure of the test involves the clinician passively assessing the patient's range of hip flexion with an extended knee, in supine. An expected positive result is a reduction of the available range of hip flexion on the affected side. The test may also reproduce the patient's symptoms.

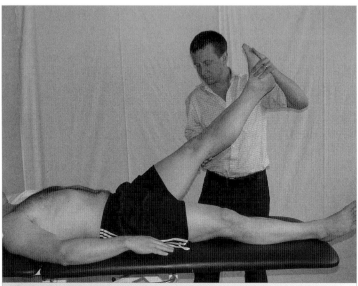

Fig 10.1 Straight leg raise: The clinician flexes the hip while keeping the knee in extension, and monitors the patient's symptoms.

PROCEDURE

Patient: The patient is positioned in supine on a plinth.

Clinician: Standing on the side of the patient to be tested, facing the patient, the clinician grasps the calf just proximal to the heel with one hand and maintains full knee extension with the other hand. The clinician passively raises the leg to the point of limitation, this being resistance to hip flexion (Fig. 10.1). The clinician notes the degree of hip flexion available and the subsequent response to the patient's symptoms. The clinician has the option to add any of the sensitizing movements. Additional sensitizing manoeuvres of ankle dorsiflexion, hip adduction, hip internal rotation and passive neck flexion may be applied. The clinician notes the result and proceeds to test the opposite side.

FINDINGS

Positive result: A degree of hip flexion available on the affected leg below 30°, with or without pain, may suggest a possible prolapsed intervertebral lumbar disc or a highly sensitized sciatic nerve. A degree of hip flexion available on the affected leg between 30° and 70° may suggest a sensitized sciatic nerve. A bilateral reduced straight leg raise may suggest a central neurodynamic problem, which may indicate more serious pathology.

Negative result: No limitation to movement; normal ranges are between 70° and 120°.

SLUMP TEST

The slump test is designed to test the neurodynamics or the sensitivity of the sciatic nerve and the spinal cord. The procedure of the test involves the clinician positioning the patient into a slumped posture and adding sensitizing manoeuvres of the cervical spine and/or lower limb. An expected positive result is a reproduction of the patient's symptoms and a potential loss of range of one of the sensitizing manoeuvres.

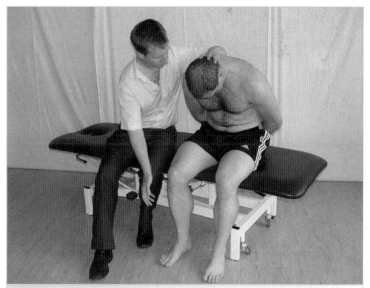

Fig 10.2   Slump test: The patient slumps from a sitting position. The clinician lightly holds the patient in position and monitors the patient's symptoms.

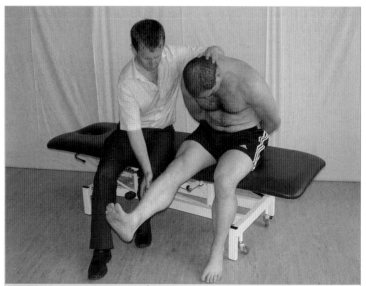

Fig 10.3 Slump test: The patient extends one knee and reports any change in symptoms.

PROCEDURE

Patient: The patient is positioned in sitting, feet flat on the floor, hands held lightly behind their back.

Clinician: The clinician sits alongside the patient and asks the patient to adopt a slump position by taking their chin to their chest and slumping from the spine (Fig. 10.2). The clinician can lightly hold the patient in this position. The clinician asks the patient to extend one knee and notes the range of knee extension and any reported change in the patient's symptoms (Fig. 10.3). The additional sensitizing manoeuvre of ankle dorsiflexion may be applied, From this position the clinician can remove or add any aspect of the position and interpret the findings accordingly.

FINDINGS

Positive result: Reproduction of the patient's symptoms and/or limitation of movement during any aspect of the position may suggest a sensitivity of the sciatic nerve and/or the central nervous system.

Negative result: No reproduction of symptoms and no limitation to movement.

PRONE KNEE BEND

The prone knee bend is designed to test the neurodynamics or the sensitivity of the femoral nerve. The procedure of the test involves the clinician passively assessing the patient's range of knee flexion with the patient positioned in supine. An expected positive result is a reproduction of the patient's symptoms and/or reduction of the available range of knee flexion on the affected side.

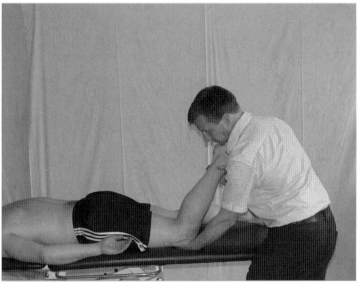

Fig 10.4 Prone knee bend: The clinician places a hand under the knee joint and ensures the pelvis is level.

PROCEDURE
Patient: The patient is positioned in prone on a plinth.
Clinician: Standing on the side of the patient to be tested, the clinician places one hand under the knee to ensure hip extension (Fig. 10.4). The clinician grasps the lower leg around the ankle joint and passively flexes the knee, and notes any reported change in symptoms and any loss of range (Fig. 10.5).

FINDINGS
Positive result: Reproduction of the patient's symptoms and/ or limitation of movement during the addition of knee flexion may suggest a sensitivity of the femoral nerve.

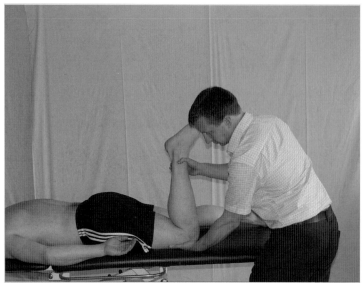

Fig 10.5   Prone knee bend: The clinician slowly flexes the patient's knee and monitors the patient's symptoms.

Negative result: No reproduction of the symptoms and no limitation to movement.

UPPER LIMB TENSION TEST 1

The upper limb tension test 1 (ULTT 1) is designed to test the neurodynamics or the sensitivity of the brachial plexus, predominantly the median nerve within the upper limb. The procedure of the test involves the clinician passively positioning the upper limb and cervical spine with a series of sensitizing manoeuvres. An expected positive result is a reproduction of the patient's symptoms and/or reduction of available range of movements on the affected side.

PROCEDURE

Patient: The patient is in supine on the plinth.

Clinician: The clinician is standing alongside the patient on the side to be tested, facing the patient. The clinician is supporting the patient's arm, with one hand under their elbow and the other at the hand. The patient's shoulder is positioned in slight abduction, their elbow in 90° flexion, forearm in pronation, wrist in neutral and fingers in extension (Fig. 10.6). The clinician then

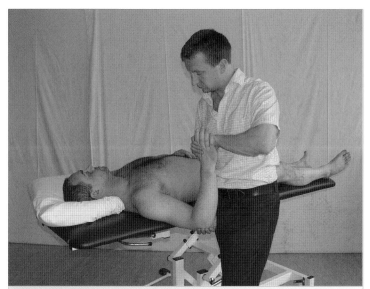

Fig 10.6   ULTT 1: Starting position.

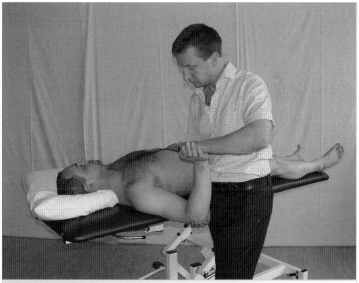

Fig 10.7   ULTT 1: Wrist extension.

applies the following manoeuvres: wrist extension (Fig. 10.7), forearm supination (Fig. 10.8), elbow extension (Fig. 10.9), shoulder lateral rotation (Fig. 10.10) and shoulder abduction (Fig. 10.11).

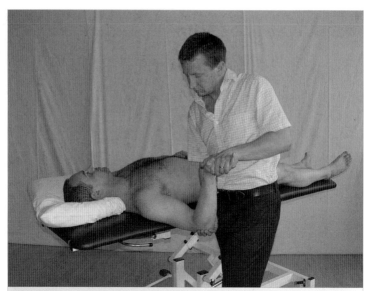

Fig 10.8   ULTT 1: Forearm supination.

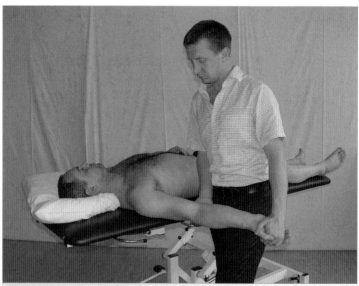

Fig 10.9   ULTT 1: Elbow extension.

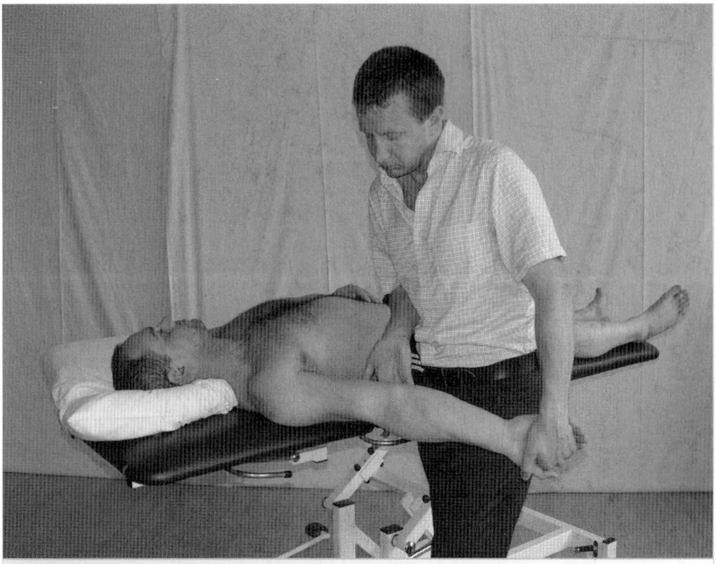

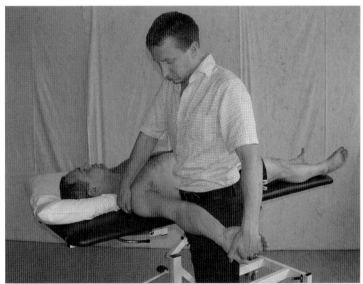

Fig 10.10   ULTT 1: Shoulder lateral rotation.

Fig 10.11   ULTT 1: Shoulder abduction.

FINDINGS

Positive result: Reproduction of the patient's symptoms and/ or limitation of movement during any of the manoeuvres may suggest a sensitization of the median nerve.

Negative result: No reproduction of the symptoms and no limitation to the movement.

UPPER LIMB TENSION TEST 2a

The upper limb tension test 2a (ULTT 2a) is designed to test the neurodynamics or the sensitivity of the brachial plexus, predominantly the median nerve within the upper limb. The procedure of the test involves the clinician passively positioning the upper limb and cervical spine with a series of sensitizing manoeuvres. An expected positive result is a reproduction of the patient's symptoms and/ or reduction of available range of movements on the affected side.

PROCEDURE

Patient: The patient is in supine on a plinth.

Clinician: The clinician is standing alongside the patient on the side to be tested, facing down the plinth. The clinician is supporting the patient's arm, with one hand under their elbow and the other at the hand. The patient's shoulder is positioned in neutral, their elbow in 90° flexion, forearm in neutral, wrist in neutral and fingers in slight flexion (Fig. 10.12). The clinician then applies the following manoeuvres: shoulder girdle depression (Fig. 10.13), elbow extension (Fig. 10.14), shoulder lateral rotation (Fig. 10.15), wrist and finger extension (Fig. 10.16) and shoulder abduction (Fig. 10.17).

FINDINGS

Positive result: Reproduction of the patient's symptoms and/ or limitation of movement during any of the manoeuvres may suggest a sensitization of the median nerve.

Negative result: No reproduction of the symptoms and no limitation to the movement.

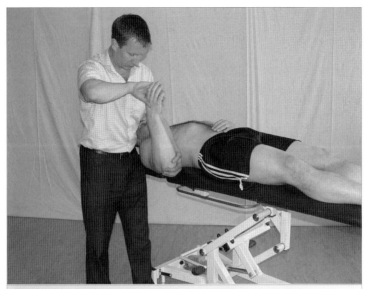

Fig 10.12   ULTT 2a: Starting position.

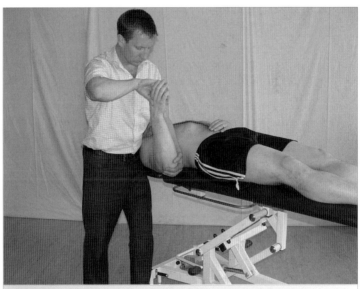

Fig 10.13   ULTT 2a: Shoulder girdle depression applied with clinician's hip.

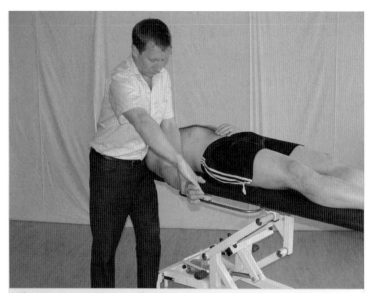

Fig 10.14   ULTT 2a: Elbow extension.

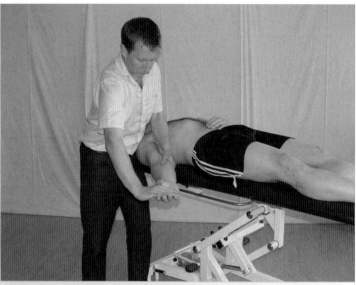

Fig 10.15   ULTT 2a: Shoulder lateral rotation.

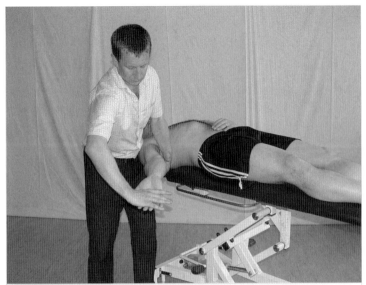

Fig 10.16   ULTT 2a: Wrist and finger extension.

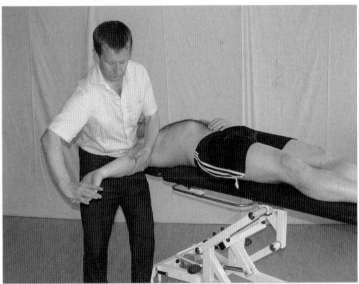

Fig 10.17   ULTT 2a: Shoulder abduction.

UPPER LIMB TENSION TEST 2b

The upper limb tension test 2b (ULTT 2b) is designed to test the neurodynamics or the sensitivity of the brachial plexus, predominantly the radial nerve within the upper limb. The procedure of the test involves the clinician passively positioning the upper limb and cervical spine with a series of sensitizing manoeuvres. An expected positive result is a reproduction of the patient's symptoms and/or reduction of available range of movements on the affected side.

PROCEDURE

Patient: The patient is in supine on the plinth.

Clinician: The clinician is standing alongside the patient on the side to be tested, facing down the plinth. The clinician is supporting the patient's arm, with one hand under their elbow and the other at the wrist. The patient's shoulder is positioned in neutral and slight abduction, their elbow in 90° flexion, forearm in neutral, wrist and fingers in flexion (Fig. 10.18). The clinician then applies the following manoeuvres: shoulder girdle depression (Fig. 10.19), elbow extension (Fig. 10.20), shoulder medial rotation (Fig. 10.21), and wrist and finger flexion (Fig. 10.22).

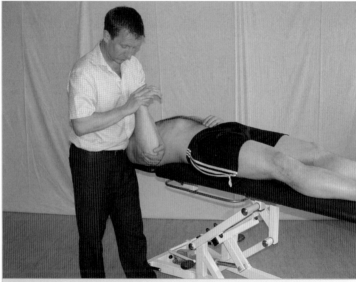

Fig 10.18   ULTT 2b: Starting position.

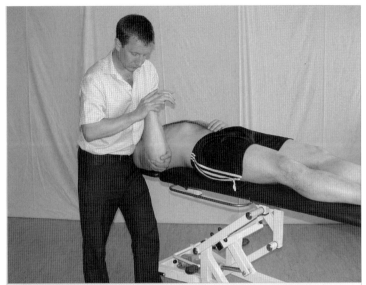

Fig 10.19   ULTT 2b: Shoulder girdle depression applied with clinician's hip.

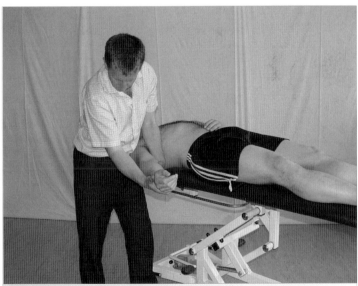

Fig 10.20   ULTT 2b: Elbow extension.

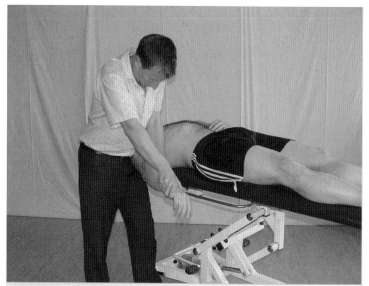

Fig 10.21   ULTT 2b: Shoulder medial rotation.

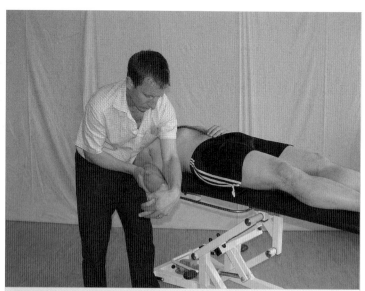

Fig 10.22   ULTT 2b: Wrist and finger flexion.

FINDINGS
Positive result: Reproduction of the patient's symptoms and/ or limitation of movement during any of the manoeuvres may suggest a sensitization of the radial nerve.

Negative result: No reproduction of the symptoms and no limitation to the movement.

UPPER LIMB TENSION TEST 3

The upper limb tension test 3 (ULTT 3) is designed to test the neurodynamics or the sensitivity of the brachial plexus, predominantly the ulnar nerve within the upper limb. The procedure of the test involves the clinician passively positioning the upper limb and cervical spine with a series of sensitizing manoeuvres. An expected positive result is a reproduction of the patient's symptoms and/or reduction of available range of movements on the affected side.

PROCEDURE
Patient: The patient is in supine on the plinth.

Clinician: The clinician is standing alongside the patient on the side to be tested, facing the patient. The clinician is supporting the patient's arm, with one hand under their elbow and the other at the hand. The patient's shoulder is positioned in neutral, their elbow in 90° flexion, forearm in pronation, wrist in neutral and fingers in extension (Fig. 10.23). The clinician then applies the

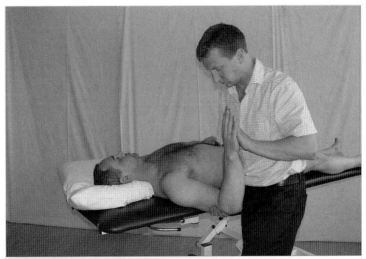

Fig 10.23   ULTT 3: Starting position.

following manoeuvres: wrist extension (Fig. 10.24), forearm pronation (Fig. 10.25), elbow flexion (Fig. 10.26), shoulder lateral rotation (Fig. 10.27), shoulder girdle depression (Fig. 10.28) and shoulder abduction (Fig. 10.29).

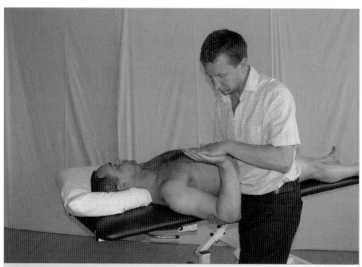

Fig 10.24　ULTT 3: Wrist extension.

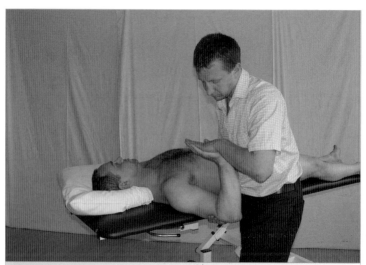

Fig 10.25　ULTT 3: Foream pronation.

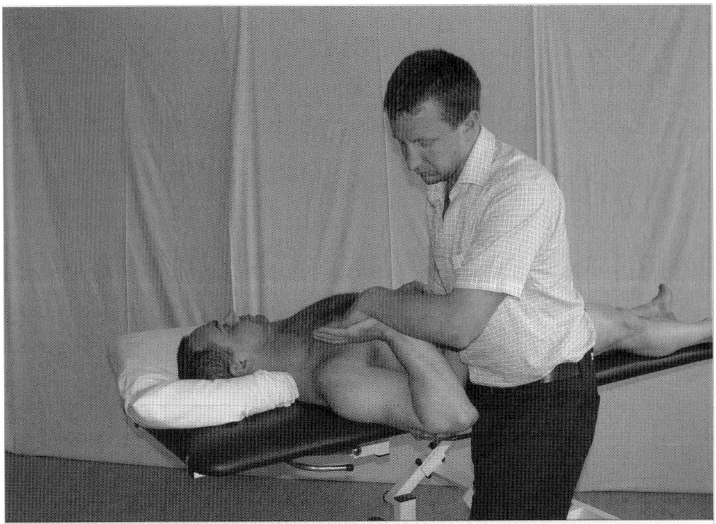

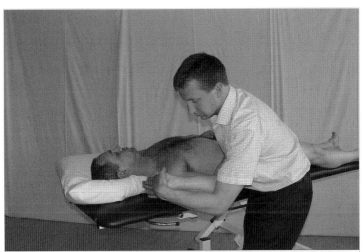

Fig 10.26   ULTT 3: Elbow flexion.

Fig 10.27   ULTT 3: Shoulder lateral rotation.

FINDINGS

Positive result: Reproduction of the patient's symptoms and/ or limitation of movement during any of the manoeuvres may suggest a sensitization of the ulnar nerve.

Negative result: No reproduction of the symptoms and no limitation to the movement.

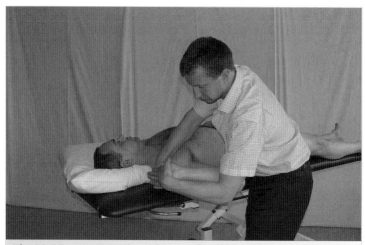

Fig 10.28   ULTT 3: Shoulder girdle depression.

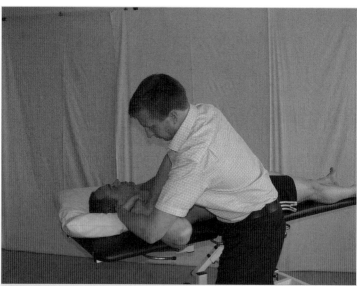

Fig 10.29   ULTT 3: Shoulder abduction.

Table 10.1 Sensitivity and specificity values of upper limb tension test

Author	Aim of study	Design	Sensitivity	Specificity
Rubinstein et al (2007)	Assessment of the diagnostic accuracy of provocative tests of the neck for diagnosis of cervical radiculopathy	Systematic review of six studies that met the selection criteria	Range 72–97%	Range 11–33%

REFERENCES

Butler D 2000 The sensitive nervous system. Noigroup Publications, Adelaide, Australia

Rubinstein S, Pool J, van Tulder M et al 2007 A systematic review of the diagnostic accuracy of provocative tests of the neck for diagnosing cervical radiculopathy. European Spine Journal 16(3): 307–319

Shacklock M 2005 Clinical neurodynamics. Elsevier, Edinburgh

Index